THE NEUMAN SYSTEMS MODEL AND NURSING EDUCATION:

Teaching Strategies and Outcomes

EDITED BY LOIS LOWRY

Sigma Theta Tau International
550 West North Street
Indianapolis, Indiana 46202

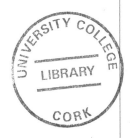

Sigma Theta Tau International
Publishing Director: Jeff Burnham
Book Acquisitions Editor: Fay L. Bower, DNSc, FAAN
Graphic Designer: Jason Reuss
Proofreader: Linda Canter

For other publications contact:
Sigma Theta Tau International
550 West North Street
Indianapolis, IN 46202
1-888-634-7575
FAX (317) 634-8188
www.nursingsociety.org/publications

ISBN: 0-9656391-5-0

Printed in the United States of America

Views expressed herein are not necessarily
those of Sigma Theta Tau International.

03 04 05 / 98765432

Table of Contents

Contributors

Sarah J. Beckman, RN, MSN
Associate Professor
Indiana University-Purdue University
Fort Wayne, IN

Sanna Boxley-Harges, RN, MA
Associate Professor
Indiana University-Purdue University
Fort Wayne, IN

Cheryl Bruick-Sorge, RN, MA
Associate Professor
Indiana University-Purdue University
Fort Wayne, IN

Priscilla Busch, RN, EdD
Associate Professor
St. Anselm College
Manchester, NH

Nahn Joo Chang, RNC, MSN
Assistant Professor
Lander University
Greenwood, SC

Bronwynne C. Evans, RN, PhD
Director of Nursing
Yakima Valley Community College
Yakima, WA

Judith Eichenaur, RN, MSN
Associate Professor
Indiana University-Purdue University
Fort Wayne, IN

Donna L. Forrest, RN, MSN
Instructor
Santa Fe Community College
Gainesville, FL

Filomena C. Flores, RN, PhD
Professor
California State University
Fresno, CA

Barbara T. Freese, RN, EdD, FRCNA
Professor and Dean
School of Nursing
Lander University
Greenwood, SC

Janet S. Hassell, MA, MS, FNP
Former Faculty
Lander University
Greenwood, SC

Contributors
(continued)

Opal A. Freiburger, RN, EdD
Associate Professor
Indiana University-Purdue University .
Fort Wayne, IN

Lois W. Lowry, RN, DNSc
Associate Professor
University of South Florida
Tampa, FL

Martha H. Lynch, RN, EdD
Associate Professor
St. Anselm College
Manchester, NH

Grace G. Newsome, FNP, EdD
LINC Coordinator
Georgia Hospital Association
Marietta, GA

Patricia R. Nuttall, RN, PhD, CPNP
Associate Professor
California State University
Fresno, CA

Carol J. Scales, RN, PhD
Assistant Professor
Lander University
Greenwood, SC

Victoria Strickland Seng, RN, PhD
Associate Professor and Chair
University of Tennessee at Martin
Martin, TN

Eleanor M. Stittich, RN, BSNE
M. Litt., Professor Emerita
California State University
Fresno, CA

Rita Sutherland, ARNP, MSN
Coordinator of Nursing Programs
Santa Fe Community College
Gainesville, FL

Kathryn C. Wood, RN, PhD
Associate Professor and Chair
State University of New York
Brockport, NY

Ann R. Weitzel, RN, MS
Assistant Professor
State University of New York
Brockport, NY

Foreword

Betty Neuman, RN, PhD, FAAN
Theorist, Consultant, Counselor

This significant work reflects the growing concern of educators about how to appropriately educate the beginning nurse. There is a dearth of literature on curricular planning, teaching strategies, and longitudinal evaluation illustrating the use of nursing models for basic nursing education programs.

The monograph fulfills the longstanding need for sharing specific processes used by experienced nurse educators in educational programming with the Neuman Systems Model. How exciting it is to learn of the many creative teaching strategies used by these nurse educators! They are to be commended for sharing their success to benefit both novice and experienced educators in this challenging era of curricular revolution. Many of these processes could enhance the application of other models, as well. It has long been my view that beginning level nurse education programs should be based on nursing models so that students can benefit from knowing the "big picture" and learning important nursing concepts that can maximize future learning activities.

The unit on evaluation provides evidence that curricula based on the Neuman Systems Model process are efficient and effective. Studies indicate that graduates do integrate concepts and process into their generalist and advanced practice roles.

Many of the authors have contributed to the literature through three editions of the Neuman Systems Model book, journal publications, and presentations of their work at biennial Neuman Systems Model Symposia and other conferences. Their work, as presented in this monograph will provide important direction and educational strategies for the many nurse educators throughout the world who have expressed a need for specific information. The processes used will be appreciated by many.

In establishing the first Neuman Systems Model-based Associate Degree in Nursing program, Dr. Lowry deserves special commendation for her early vision in understanding the need for the development of a unique longitudinal evaluation protocol. She has well validated her philosophy of the importance of model-based first educational level programming. Both she and her colleagues have made a major contribution to theoretical nursing education.

Dr. Lowry has truly accepted the leadership challenge, as a longstanding supporter of the model and member of the Neuman Systems Model Trustees, to promote use of the model for nursing education and practice now and into the 21st century.

The monograph should have far-reaching effects by contributing specific educational programming directives and by increasing visibility for greater model utility in diverse cultures worldwide.

Acknowledgements
Lois W. Lowry

It is with deep respect and gratitude for the contributors to this project that I present this monograph. Each author has shared her creative ideas and educational expertise so that other educators might benefit from her experiences. My hope is that this book will lead to subsequent publications that can inform and inspire educators as they continue in their dedication to student learning. I am grateful to my typist, Marie Taylor, who dedicated many hours to actualize my dream.

Special thanks and recognition to:
Betty Neuman, my inspiration and friend, who encouraged me to undertake this project. She is a lady whose vision and dedication to students has fostered the creation and continuation of the Neuman Systems Model for nurses yesterday, today, and tomorrow.

Jacqueline Fawcett, my first theory teacher, who introduced me to the creative worlds of theorists and has continued to challenge me to extend the science of nursing through scholarly analysis and evaluation of nursing theories.

Rosalie Mirenda, who served as my first mentor.

The faculty of Neuman College, who were the source of knowledge for the faculty of Cecil Community College as we accepted the challenge to develop, implement, and evaluate a Neuman-based curriculum.

The Neuman Systems Model Trustees, Inc., who provide a continuing support network for future visioning and implementation of the model.

> "Throughout centuries
> There were those
> Who took first steps
> Down new roads
> Armed with nothing
> But their vision."
> —Ayn Rand

Preface

Lois W. Lowry
NSM Trustee

This monograph is a collection of writings by educators who have used the Neuman Systems Model as a framework for curricula and courses in associate, baccalaureate, and master's degree programs over the past 10 years. The purpose of the monograph is to share successful teaching strategies, evaluation instruments, and processes developed by educators from various Neuman Systems Model-based nursing education programs. Inherent in the purpose are the beliefs that model-based programs enhance critical thinking of nursing students and that educational evaluation can assist educators to determine the credibility of nursing models.

Each chapter of the monograph was written by faculty from different colleges or universities that have Neuman Systems Model-based programs. Each author presents either unique teaching strategies that have enhanced student learning or an educational evaluation process. This approach differs from other publications in that strategies and instruments cited in this monograph are specifically related to the Neuman Systems Model. Educators who base their programs or courses on other conceptual models could, however, use the strategies and examples in this monograph as blueprints for teaching and evaluation.

In recent years, a trend in nursing education has been to move from curricula based on Tylerian-behaviorist principles toward a paradigm that values teacher and student interactions. This contemporary educational process shifts the focus from training to education, from strict content objectives to critical thinking strategies, and from lecture to student-teacher dialogues and socratic questioning. This monograph describes how nursing programs and courses are developed from an educative-interpretive paradigm.

Unit I sets the direction for the monograph. Chapter 1 provides an overview of the Neuman Systems Model and describes how Neuman Systems Model-based programs can be developed from both the Tylerian-behaviorist and the educative-interpretive paradigms. Chapter 2 presents an overview of strategies that integrate the model, critical thinking, and cooperative learning. Chapter 3 includes an historical overview of evaluation in education, popular evaluative models, and their use in Neuman Systems Model-based programs.

Unit II presents eight chapters about teaching/learning strategies that have been successful in Neuman Systems Model-based courses and programs at the associate, baccalaureate, and master's degree levels. Chapters 4 and 5 explain how critical thinking strategies are incorporated in associate and baccalaureate degree programs. Chapter 6 presents useful strategies for learning concepts related to family and community as client. Chapter 7 provides a creative approach to teaching a nursing issues course. Chapter 8 presents an example of teaching culturally safe care for Korean-Americans. Chapter 9 provides an overview of the content of a community health course in a baccalaureate program and strategies to enhance learning. Chapter 10 presents an innovative application of primary prevention interventions within an Associate of Science curriculum. Chapter 11 describes an advanced nurse curriculum based upon the Neuman Systems Model.

Unit III presents seven chapters that address evaluation processes and outcomes of Neuman-based courses and programs. Chapter 12 introduces Guba's model and the process of evaluation at Yakima Valley Community College. Chapter 13 presents clinical evaluation instruments from the Nursing Department of the University of Tennessee at Martin. Chapter 14 describes how outcome evaluation data are collected for making decisions about program effectiveness. Chapters 15 and 16 present end-of-program evaluation studies that used the Lowry-Jopp Neuman Model Evaluation Instrument. These are the first documented studies of the efficacy of the Neuman Systems Model as a curriculum framework. Chapter 17 presents an explanation of how faculty interest in the model can be developed and renewed. Chapter 18 concludes the monograph with a discussion of Neuman Systems Model values that influence use of the model throughout the world.

Unit I: Charting the Direction

"A good mind is like a good parachute;
it only works when it is open."
—Anonymous

Preparing nurse graduates for a changing health care system requires that educators think creatively and innovate boldly. Educators must compare old educational paradigms with newer ones to find a "good fit" that will achieve the educational goals for preparing students for the future. Chapters in Unit I provide theoretical background for the strategies described in Unit II and the evaluation processes described in Unit III.

Chapter 1
Creative Teaching and Effective Evaluation
Lois W. Lowry

Nurse educators have been challenged for more than 20 years to develop curricula based upon conceptual models for nursing education programs. The primary advantage of teaching and learning from a model is that the model sets the direction and provides the world view for the organization of content that is taught and the evaluation of the learning that takes place. Nurse educators frequently use models in education that are borrowed uncritically from other disciplines (e.g., medical model, various psychological and sociological models, occasionally organizational and economic models). Nursing models, on the other hand, focus attention on clients who are recipients of nursing care. The Neuman Systems Model has been one of the most popular nursing models selected by educators as the conceptual framework for associate and baccalaureate degree programs. A few master's programs use the Neuman model as the basis for advanced practice curricula; others have selected the model to guide specific course or clinical practicum development when a systems perspective is appropriate.

The contributors to this monograph believe in the efficacy of developing curricula from nursing conceptual models. When educators accept the challenge to develop a new curriculum or to revise an old one from the viewpoint of a nursing conceptual model, they may find sparse information in the literature that could assist them in developing courses and evaluation instruments. Thus, educators in model-based nursing programs are left to develop both their teaching strategies to enhance student understanding of model constructs and their instruments to test learning. If examples of unique strategies could be communicated to other educators, the burden of course development could be eased. Educators in current model-based programs tend to use strategies that reflect the goals of the new paradigm for curriculum development and teaching; namely critical thinking, contextual, syntactical, and inquiry learning. Revised accreditation criteria require documentation of critical thinking within associate and basic baccalaureate curricula; whereas, critical thinking, analysis, and synthesis are the hallmarks of advanced practice nursing programs. Thus, the importance of a forum for sharing innovative strategies among educators is documented.

If we believe that nursing models contribute to more effective teaching and learning and that practicing from a model provides more comprehensive care and high-quality outcomes for clients, then we must demonstrate the efficacy of models through evaluation of model-based programs. There is little published evidence that graduates from model-based programs continue to practice according to model perspectives upon graduation, although faculty in these programs would attest to their efficacy. Educators in model-based programs with strong evaluation components must share their findings so that others have a basis for making informed decisions about the use of models in guiding curriculum development. Chapter 1 sets the direction for the monograph by explicating the versatility, breadth, and flexibility of the Neuman Systems Model as an example of a nursing paradigm that is appropriate for curriculum development and evaluation within the behaviorist and educative-interpretive paradigms.

A Nursing Paradigm

The Neuman Systems Model is one of the four models most often used for nursing curriculum development since the early 1980s (Lewis & Koertvelgessy, 1989). Many examples of the use of the Neuman Systems Model in associate, baccalaureate, and master's programs are summarized by Fawcett (1994) and presented in chapters in the three editions of Neuman's (1982, 1989, 1995) books. Programs in many schools from across the country are based on the Neuman Systems Model. Concepts of the model that appeal to faculty who are developing or revising curricula include principles of systems thinking, a wholistic view of clients, and emphasis on the reciprocity of nurse-client interactions. A familiar vocabulary and an emphasis on stress and its effects are also concepts that contribute to understanding the model. The concepts of primary, secondary, and tertiary prevention as intervention provide an action plan for nurses that can assist in assessment, intervention, and evaluation of outcomes.

Neuman initially proposed the model for graduate students in order to provide unity or a focal point for learning (Neuman, 1995, p. 674). Neuman based her conceptualizations on knowledge of general system theory, which proposed a science of wholes and wholeness that would provide a possible approach toward the unification of science (Von Bertalanffy, 1968). Living, open systems, as defined by Von Bertalanffy (1968), exchange energy with the environment to maintain themselves and develop a steady state. Based on systems principles, Neuman's model proposes wholism as "optimizing a dynamic yet stable interrelationship of spirit, mind, and body of the client in a constantly changing environment and society" (Neuman, 1995, p. 10).

Neuman's client system, which can be a person, family, group, or community, is composed of five variables—physiological, psychological, sociocutural, developmental, and spiritual. These variables interact dynamically to keep the system stable. The strength and interaction of the variables determines the degree of resistance the client system has to stressors or forces from the environment that threaten to disturb system equilibrium. Neuman identifies three environments: an *internal environment* within the client system that is a source of intra-personal stressors, an *external environment* outside the client system that is a source of inter- and extra-personal stressors, and a *created environment*. The created environment is developed unconsciously by the client system as a protective coping mechanism against stressors. The time, nature, and intensity of one or more stressors have the potential for reaction with the client system depending on the client's condition and past coping behaviors.

Neuman depicts the client system as a series of concentric circles surrounding a *central core* that consists of basic survival factors, genetic characteristics, and strengths and weaknesses of system parts. The outermost circle, the *flexible line of defense,* serves as a protective buffer for clients' normal state. It is conceptualized as an accordion-like mechanism that expands outward when a client is experiencing high levels of energy that preserve and enhance system integrity and contracts toward the *normal line of defense* when less energy is available. As the flexible line of defense draws closer to the normal line of defense, less protection is available against stressor effects. The normal line of defense is the second concentric circle that represents what the client has become, the state to which the client has evolved over time, and the usual wellness level. It represents the stability and integrity of the system that has developed over time, including life-style factors, coping patterns, and developmental, cultural, and spiritual factors. It is also dynamic but expands and contracts to a lesser extent than the flexible line of defense.

The innermost circles that surround the core are *lines of resistance* such as the body's immune system, coping mechanisms, and spiritual resources. These lines of resistance are activated when environmental stressors break through the flexible and normal lines of defense, and they assist in reversing the reaction to stressors. If effective, the client system begins to *reconstitute,* leading to a return to a healthy state. If ineffective, the system experiences energy depletion and, ultimately, death will occur.

The goal of nursing is to keep the client system stable through accurate assessment of stressor reactions followed by initiation of interventions that can promote wellness. The interventions include primary, secondary, and tertiary preventions. *Primary prevention* is aimed at strengthening the flexible line of defense by reducing stress and risk factors. Usually primary prevention begins before stressor invasion occurs.

Secondary prevention is initiated after a reaction to a stressor has already occurred and the lines of resistance are activated. Nurse actions include identification of stressors and assessment of the degree of reaction to stressor(s). Then interventions are selected which strengthen the lines of resistance. *Tertiary prevention* begins following the initiation of secondary prevention interventions after some degree of system stability occurs. *Tertiary prevention* interventions are aimed at readaptation, reeducation, and maintenance of stability to prevent further stressor reaction or regression. All existing resources, external and internal, are considered to support existing strengths and to conserve client system energy. All three prevention-as-intervention modalities can be used with any client system resulting in synergistic benefits. The ultimate goal is to attain, maintain, or retain system stability resulting in optimal health for clients (Neuman, 1995).

The original diagram (**Figure 1.1**) that includes all the major model concepts has not been altered through the years, although Neuman has elaborated on the concept of environment and the variable "spirituality" in the third edition of her book (Neuman, 1995). The basic assumptions of the model, now viewed as propositions, explicate the interrelationships of the model concepts (**Table 1.1**). Readers requiring more in-depth information about the model are referred to chapters in the three editions of *The Neuman Systems Model* by Dr. Betty Neuman (1982, 1989, 1995).

Table 1.1: Propositions of the Neuman Systems Model.

1. Although each individual client or group as a client system is unique, each system is a composite of common known factors or innate characteristics within a normal, given range of response contained within a basic structure.

2. Many known, unknown, and universal environmental stressors exist. Each differs in its potential for disturbing a client's usual stability level, or normal line of defense. The particular interrelationships of client variables-physiological, psychological, sociocultural, developmental, and spiritual-at any point in time can affect the degree to which a client is protected by the flexible line of defense against possible reaction to a single stressor or a combination of stressors.

3. Each individual client/client system has evolved a normal range of response to the environment that is referred to as a normal line of defense, or usual wellness/stability state. It represents change over time through coping with diverse stress encounters. The normal line of defense can be used as a standard from which to measure health deviation.

4. When the cushioning, accordion-like effect of the flexible line of defense is no longer capable of protecting the client/client system against an environmental stressor, the stressor breaks through the normal line of defense. The interrelationships of variables-physiological, psychological, sociocultural, developmental, and spiritual-determine the nature and degree of system reaction or possible reaction to the stressor.

5. The client, whether in a state of wellness or illness, is a dynamic composite of the interrelationships of variables-physiological, psychological, sociocultural, developmental, and spiritual. Wellness is on a continuum of available energy to support the system in an optimal state of system stability.

6. Implicit within each client system are internal resistance factors known as lines of resistance, which function to stabilize and return the client to the usual wellness state (normal line of defense) or possibly to a higher level of stability following an environmental stressor reaction.

7. Primary prevention relates to general knowledge that is applied in client assessment and intervention in identification and reduction or mitigation of possible or actual risk factors associated with environmental stressors to prevent possible reaction. The goal of health promotion is included in primary prevention.

8. Secondary prevention relates to symptomatology following a reaction to stressors, appropriate ranking of intervention priorities, and treatment to reduce their noxious effects.

9. Tertiary prevention relates to the adjustive processes taking place as reconstitution begins and maintenance factors move the client back in a circular manner toward primary prevention.

10. The client as a system is in dynamic, constant energy exchange with the environment.

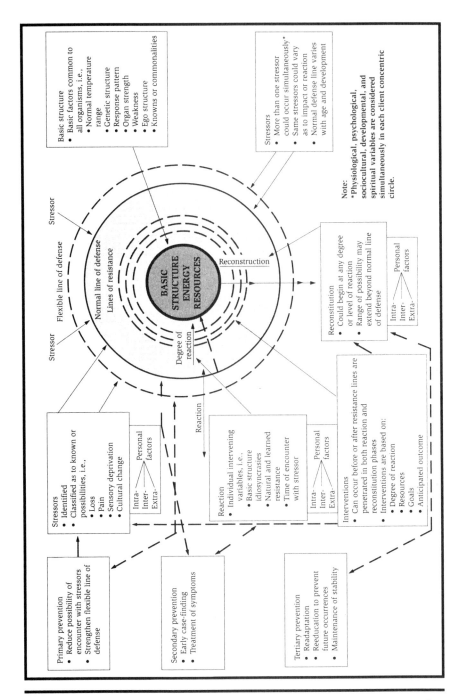

Figure 1.1: The Neuman Systems Model 1989. (From Neuman, B: The Neuman Systems Model, 2nd ed., East Norwalk, CT: Appleton & Lange).

Educational Paradigms

Educators who choose a nursing model as the framework for organizing curriculum content must also select an educational paradigm to guide curriculum development and teaching-learning strategies. One can safely assume that most of the Neuman-based curricula designed in the late 1970s to early 1980s used the behaviorist paradigm. The curriculum often followed a blueprint created by Bower (1982) that was consistent with model constructs and gave direction for generating objectives, content, and organization. The Neuman Model provided the organization, concepts, and philosophical underpinnings for the curriculum, and the Bower blueprint illustrated how the curriculum should be designed. Faculty in some programs created their own curriculum design. In such instances, faculty immersed themselves into the model, seeking to internalize the concepts and their definitions, while reconciling the faculty's philosophies of person, environment, nursing, and health with Neuman's philosophy (Lowry & Jopp, 1989; Mirenda, 1996). Although baccalaureate programs were the first to adopt the Neuman model as a curriculum framework, associate degree programs began to follow the trend in the 1980s. To a lesser degree master's level programs found the model appropriate. There is at least one innovative Advanced Nurse Practitioner program—in Fresno, California—based on Neuman's framework.

A new curriculum paradigm has evolved—the educative/professional model—in which nurses are educated rather than trained; this model is better and more appropriate than the Tylerian model. In the Tylerian approach, the philosophy of nursing education was pragmatic, highly structured, and empirical. Teaching was by rules and procedures that produced efficient technical nurses but did not lead students to a better understanding of people and how they cope with health and illness (Bevis & Watson, 1989). Behaviorists tend to be preoccupied with "what to teach," resulting in a distorted relationship between students and their worlds (Moccia, 1989). Professional education requires more emphasis on the "how" of teaching rather than the "what." The process of education wholistically reconciles individuals and their world by encouraging learning activities that are egalitarian and interactive (Gray, 1984). Education for the future focuses on soul and process. It emphasizes "uncovering the entire complexity of real connections between apparently unrelated phenomena, and in that uncovering is the creation of new connections, new possibilities" (Moccia, 1989, p. xi). In no discipline is this educational philosophy more important than in nursing. Nurses must know themselves and their world in order to learn to know others and their worlds. Through this learning process, nurses will be able to use themselves as vehicles for client growth and empowerment.

To advance nursing through educative learning, nurse educators are challenged to implement the new paradigm in curriculum development so that graduates are skilled, compassionate, scholar-clinicians. The central thesis of the new paradigm is that "curriculum is the interactions and traditions that occur between and among students and teachers with the intent that learning occur" (Bevis & Watson, 1989, p. 5). Active learning between teachers and students is the foremost strategy to be used in the classroom, and the Neuman Systems Model provides the content framework through which students and teachers exchange ideas about people, their stressors, and reactions to stress requiring nursing interventions.

Among classroom teachers there is a pervasive belief that "we are all good teachers" (Eison & Bonwell, 1993). Thus, little incentive exists in the minds of many faculty to try new approaches. In fact, faculty often view change as just "more work" added to an already overloaded schedule. On the other hand, faculty who perceive education as an immersion of the whole person into the endeavor and who perceive change as both consistent with existing values and a means toward better methods are more likely to adopt innovations. Knowledge about alternative teaching strategies and designs can also reduce faculty resistance to change. Faculty who accept the challenge to develop a model-based curriculum have already demonstrated their openness to innovation. Therefore, even if a Neuman-based curriculum were originally designed from a behaviorist perspective, the model itself is broad and comprehensive enough to accommodate the learning typology of the new paradigm.

Faculty who truly wish to educate rather than train must focus on fostering learning maturity through modification of teacher-student relationships (Bevis & Watson, 1989). This implies that faculty know what types of learning strategies promote learning maturity and will select modalities that provide the context, content, and focus for educative learning. Bevis and Watson (1989) suggest a typology that includes contextual, syntactical, and inquiry learning. Awareness of these types of learning coupled with the use of teaching methods to enhance each type will assist students in moving toward maturity.

The Neuman Model and the Educative-Interpretive Paradigm

The Neuman Systems Model provides a flexible framework that supports the typology of context, syntax, and inquiry. For example, model definitions and assumptions suggest the context in which the practice of nursing is learned. Faculty who adopt the model as a curriculum framework usually do so after investigating several models and ultimately selecting the one with a philosophy most similar to their own basic philosophy of nursing. The Neuman Systems Model does not dictate the arrangement of curriculum content. These decisions remain with faculty. Curriculum content is presented through the language and world view of Neuman. For example, Neuman's definitions of client systems, lines of defense, stress, reaction to stress, optimal system stability, and prevention as intervention are concepts that give structure and meaning to all courses. Specific content is framed by these concepts.

Neuman believes that the role of the nurse is to "keep the client system stable through accurate assessment of actual and potential effects of environmental stressors and in assisting client adjustments required for an optimal wellness level" (Neuman, 1995, p. 34). Thus, the model provides the focus of nursing's concern, and the three prevention-as-intervention modalities suggest the actions required to reach client goals. The model, then, provides the contextual learning that enables students to think and act like nurses. The language of the model directs students' understanding of nurse-client relationships.

Use of Neuman's model promotes syntactical learning through its structure—into which data can be arranged producing meaningful wholes. The model presents the broad general relationships among concepts that can be specifically illustrated through case studies. Case studies require learners to depart from a usual or customary nursing intervention to plan for care patterned specifically for a unique client in a particular situation. Selecting cues and making inferences that can direct a plan of action is one of the imperatives of critical thinking. Students learn to act and judge on the basis of a reasoned appraisal of the situation at hand.

Neuman emphasizes that clients' perceptions of their problems, situations, or hospitalizations be considered as well as the nurse's perceptions. This emphasis legitimizes feelings and intuition as valid and important considerations of every nurse-client interaction in the processes of goal setting and achievement. One of the foci of syntactical learning is to acknowledge personal opinions and experiences. As these informal elements are integrated with the formal factual data, students learn to generate personal guides for care giving. Students are encouraged to depart from typical care plans and to create individualized goals. The extent of achievement in this type of learning influences the degree of expertise one acquires—first as a student, and then as a graduate.

The dynamic nature of the model enables personal experiences with clients to be interpreted through the theoretical principles of stress, reaction to stress, and systems thinking. Personal experiences enhance understanding of the model propositions and, in turn, the model promotes interpretation of personal experiences. This welding of theory and practice into praxis enables students to use and to trust intuition (Bevis & Watson, 1989).

The Neuman Systems Model encourages inquiry learning. Neuman creatively constructed the model from her own clinical and teaching experiences in mental health nursing and her synthesis of knowledge from several scholars. Her motivation to construct the model was a response to the expressed needs of graduate students in the School of Nursing, University of California at Los Angeles, for course content that would represent the breadth of nursing perspectives before content that emphasizes specific nursing problem areas (Neuman & Young, 1972). The model was originally developed as a "teaching aid" (Neuman, 1989, p. 456). In creating this model, Neuman generated an idea, presented a new way of configuring old ideas, visualized future possibilities, and invented a way to bring the ideas into reality for students. Inquiry learning encompasses "the art of investigation, the search for truth, the generation of theory, and the development of new ideas, dreams, and visions" (Bevis & Watson, 1989, p. 94). The development of a model is a prime example of the highest level of learning. Students of today are challenged to test Neuman's propositions; to develop hypotheses from model constructs and to test them. Research studies are imperative to validate or refute the credibility of the model.

As our world becomes increasingly complex and change accelerates, educators realize that the ability to think critically is related to success in life. They also recognize that there must be changes in modes of instruction so that students learn the tools of critical thinking. Richard Paul, a major leader in the international critical thinking movement, has identified three "waves" of research into critical thinking since the early 1970s (Paul, 1995). Each wave represents a different research agenda and emphasis in application. The first-wave theorists (1970-1980) focused on reasoning and logic, expecting college graduates to achieve minimal competence in inductive and deductive processes including an understanding of fallacies of language and thought. Courses were designed to teach logic, reasoning, and argumentation (Paul, 1995). Although the goal was comprehensive, the means to the goal were narrow, resulting in little transfer effect from the classroom to life.

Thus, the second-wave theorists (1980-1993) emerged to teach critical thinking outside the tradition of logic. These theorists represented many disciplines, including nursing, which were concerned with developing models for teaching critical thinking within a particular subject or discipline. Emphasis was placed on fostering attitudes, dispositions, and values that underlie critical thinking, so that students could translate the processes of critical thinking into the discipline and into everyday life. Unfortunately, Paul (1995) claims little effort was made to ever promote the insights from the first wave into the needs of the second. Thus, critical thinking within a specific discipline has tended to result in some disjointed and superficial results.

The third wave (1993 to present) emphasizes logical thinking that is discipline specific. Educators in Neuman-based programs claim that the model does assist students in developing critical thinking skills. Although the programs developed in the early 1980s from a behaviorist paradigm did not directly address the development of critical thinking, the model provided a context within which critical thinking could occur. As more educators adopt the new paradigm for teaching-learning, strategies for the development of critical thinking are explicitly incorporated into the program. The structure and concepts of the model, undergirded by an intellectually disciplined process of actively analyzing, synthesizing, and evaluating can achieve the goals of the third wave of critical thinking in practice and education.

In 1970, the National League for Nursing (NLN) mandated that basic nursing programs be based upon nursing frameworks. Although this is no longer required, a 1991 mandate from the NLN demands that all accredited schools specify how the program promotes and produces critical thinking skills in its graduates. Will the combination of a model-based program with an emphasis on the development of critical thinking strategies produce nurse graduates who will know how to think and how to assess their thinking? Neuman educators would answer in the affirmative. Data validating the effectiveness of model-based and, specifically, Neuman-based curricula for enhancing student learning and nursing practice are scarce, however. Few programs have attempted to validate the efficacy of the model. Data from evaluation studies are needed to support the belief.

The Neuman Model and Evaluation

Evaluation is a tool and means to determine merit or worth of progress, direction, effectiveness, and usefulness. In the behaviorist curriculum, learning objectives are written so that they may be evaluated. If a behavior is not observable or testable, it is not part of the curriculum. Educators from Neuman-based programs that follow a behaviorist model design evaluation tools based on Neuman constructs. For example, clinical evaluation tools include select behaviors that students must perform to indicate that they have assessed, planned, and evaluated client care from a Neuman perspective. A second example is client assessment tools that use Neuman concepts such as the five variables, client stressors, and reactions to stress to guide students' thinking as they collect data to plan care. The three preventions-as-interventions become the guide for the development of client interventions. Faculty then evaluate the completed assessment and care plan, not only for completeness of data, but also for how well the Neuman Model concepts have been integrated and used to plan care. The few program evaluators who conduct end-of-program evaluations also use objective items to assess the extent to which students have internalized model constructs and used them in their practice.

Evaluation in the educative-interpretive paradigm would shift emphasis from evaluating behaviors to finding ways to assess indicators of growth and learning. This paradigmatic thinking places as much importance on the students' intuition and on perceiving and judging the process of their own learning as on learning the content (Bevis & Watson, 1989). The two approaches to evaluation stem from different world views, yet can coexist in one program so long as educators are aware of the purposes of each and the ways in which they complement or contradict each other (Merton, 1975). As educators become more comfortable with viewing students as colearners and providing environments in which higher order learning (contextual, syntactical, and inquiry) can occur, they will also develop ways to evaluate these processes of learning.

How can Neuman-based curricula be evaluated from an educative-caring perspective that is congruent with the educational-interpretive paradigm? First, one must return to the philosophical foundations of the Neuman Model: wholism, gestalt, dynamic freedom, and creativity in adjusting to stressors (Neuman, 1995, p. 10). Neuman intends that the model should provide a structure that depicts parts, subparts, and their interrelationships within a whole client-environment system. Whereas use of the behaviorist-evaluative paradigm would call for assessing the parts, subparts, and behavior change of client-environment systems, the educative-interpretive paradigm would call for assessing the insights, patterns, and meanings that students gain from using the model in its entirety.

For example, the Neuman model provides for consideration of perceptual differences between caregiver and client in ways that might impede collaborative goal-setting. Each party explores ways to have a meeting of the minds so that goals can be attained. Further, the client-environment system can be viewed as an interactive whole—e.g., stressors from the environment affect clients and clients can affect the environment. Having intuition about and perceiving the mutual effects of client and environment enable students to understand wholes and to relate the parts in ways that produce meaning from the situation. This involves the ability to perceive what is significant and what is not; and then, intuiting a conclusion or an action. Teaching students to use their intuition had been an anathema to nursing until Benner's (1984) seminal work. Within the educative-interpretive paradigm, teachers would help students enhance their perceptive powers and attend to their intuition (Bevis & Watson, 1989).

The Neuman model is applicable to teacher-learner relationships as well as client-nurse relationships. In this example, students, as the center of the system, interact with teachers within the context of a teaching-learning environment. Teachers provide a climate that communicates values of care and concern for students. Students accept responsibility for a relationship that implies motivation and accountability for learning. Together, teachers and students co-create an environment in which they select goals, create learning experiences, and interpret them in ways that promote thinking and knowing.

Both teachers and learners engage with subject matter. They investigate scholarly problems. Evaluation becomes a shared student-teacher activity in which discussions elicit student meanings of their experiences. They investigate how they know and what kind of knowing they experience. Learners are in dialogue with their own learning, critiquing their work, thus progressing in learning.

The gestalt of teacher-learner interaction is congruent with Neuman's philosophy of wholeness, dynamic freedom, and creativity. The breadth of the Neuman Systems Model can help students perceive relationship patterns and meanings among the primary and secondary concepts. This is valuable learning in a time of accelerating change as the health care system becomes more complex. The Neuman model supports the educative-caring evaluative process by providing an illustration for students in which they may discover valuable relationships that enhance insight and awareness.

Summary

This chapter has set the direction for the monograph by describing the versatility of the Neuman model in both the behaviorist and educative-interpretive paradigms. The model's breadth and comprehensiveness provide a framework that is applicable to many situations. Sometimes the model has been at the forefront of educational trends, while at other times it has followed current trends. In either case, its utility in education is well documented. Subsequent chapters will introduce readers to creative teaching strategies used in Neuman-based programs as educators navigate a course that fosters critical thinking and inquiry learning. The final unit includes successful evaluation strategies and outcomes that demonstrate the efficacy of Neuman's model.

References

Benner, P. (1984). **From novice to expert: excellence and power in clinical nursing practice.** Menlo Park, CA: Addison-Wesley.

Bevis, E.M., & Watson, J. (1989). Toward a caring curriculum: a new pedagogy for nursing (Pub. No. 15-2278). **New York: National League for Nursing,** p. 5.

Bower, F.L. (1982). Curriculum development and the Neuman Model. In B. Neuman (Ed.), **The Neuman Systems Model: Application to nursing education and practice** (pp. 94-99). Norwalk, CT: Appleton-Century-Crofts.

Eison, J.A., & Bonwell, C.C. (1993). Recent works on using active learning strategies across the disciplines. Unpublished Manuscript (ERIC document reproduction service No. ED 364 135).

Fawcett, J. (1994). **Analysis and evaluation of conceptual models of nursing** (3rd ed.). Philadelphia: F.A. Davis.

Gray, J.G. (1984). **Re-thinking American education: A philosophy of teaching and learning** (2nd ed.). Connecticut: Wesleyan University Press.

Lewis, M., & Koertvelgessy, A. (1989). The Neuman model in nursing research. In B. Neuman (Ed.), **The Neuman Systems Model** (2nd ed.). Norwalk, CT: Appleton & Lange.

Lowry, L.W., & Jopp, M.C. (1989). An evaluation instrument for assessing an associate degree nursing curriculum based on the Neuman Systems Model. In J.P. Riehl-Sisca (Ed.), **Conceptual models for nursing practice** (pp. 73-85). Norwalk, CT: Appleton & Lange.

Merton, R.K. (1975). Structural analysis in sociology. In P. Blau (Ed.), **Approaches to the study of social structures.** New York: The Free Press.

Mirenda, R.M. (1996). The Neuman Systems Model: Description and application. In P. Winstead-Fry (Ed.), **Case studies in nursing theory** (pp. 127-166). New York: National League for Nursing.

Moccia, P. (1989). Preface. In E.M. Bevis & J. Watson (Eds.), **Toward a caring curriculum: A new pedagogy for nursing (Pub. No. 15-2278).** New York: National League for Nursing.

Neuman, B. (1982). **The Neuman Systems Model.** Norwalk, CT: Appleton-Century-Crofts.

Neuman, B. (1989). **The Neuman Systems Model** (2nd ed.). Norwalk, CT: Appleton & Lange.

Neuman, B. (1995). **The Neuman Systems Model** (3rd ed.). Norwalk. CT: Appleton & Lange.

Neuman, B., & Young, R.J. (1972). A model for teaching total person approach to patient problems. **Nursing Research, 21,** 264-269.

Paul, R. (1995). Critical thinking and the state of education today. Paper presented at the 16th International Conference on Critical Thinking, Sonoma, CA.

Von Bertalanffy, L. (1968). General Systems Theory: A critical review. In W. Buckley (Ed.), **Modern systems research for the behavioral scientist.** Chicago: Aldine Pub.

Watson, J. (1989). Transformative thinking and a caring curriculum. In E.M. Bevis & J. Watson (Eds.), **Toward a caring curriculum: A new pedagogy for nursing (Pub. No. 15-2278)** (p. 3). New York: National League for Nursing.

Chapter 2
Overview of Strategies that Integrate the Neuman Systems Model, Critical Thinking, and Cooperative Learning
Opal A. Freiburger

Educating students for the 21st century challenges educators to prepare people to function effectively in a highly complex global environment. Institutions of higher education and accrediting bodies (National League for Nursing, 1990; North Central Association of Colleges and Schools, 1992) as well as the American Association of Colleges of Nursing (1993), view evidence of critical thinking as a vital curriculum outcome measure. Critical thinking incorporates such intellectual processes as analyzing, synthesizing, and reasoning; cultivation of which requires time, effort, and practice. Thus, educators must use strategies that will provide an atmosphere in which students can develop high-level thinking abilities. A cooperative style of learning provides an environment that enhances students' ability to share information, ask questions, consider differing perspectives, and construct knowledge out of discourse. Testing and refining these abilities in the classroom multiply the number and often increase the complexity of shared experiences. These shared experiences influence and shape student actions in practice.

The Neuman Systems Model (NSM) is an excellent framework for the development of nursing curricula. The utility and flexibility of the model provide a comprehensive, dynamic structure for integrating a wholistic view of nursing content, critical-thinking skills for applying knowledge, and a cooperative learning style that promotes active participation. This chapter will provide an overview of critical thinking and cooperative learning principles as well as teaching and learning strategies appropriate for an educative-interpretive paradigm for teaching a Neuman-based nursing curriculum.

Critical Thinking

Critical thinking, as defined by Paul (1993), is the "intellectually disciplined process of actively and skillfully conceptualizing, applying, analyzing, synthesizing, and/or evaluating information gathered from, or generated by, observation, experience, reflection, reasoning, or communication as a guide to belief and action" (p. 18). A growing consensus of experts claims that teaching critical thinking extends beyond development of thinking skills to encouraging and inspiring people to cultivate lifelong use of critical thinking. Based upon the American Philosophical Association's Delphi Report (1990), the California Critical Thinking Disposition Inventory (CCTDI) was developed by Facione and Facione (1994). Seven aspects of critical thinking represented in this instrument include being (a) inquisitive (intellectual curiosity and learning desire); (b) systematic (organized, orderly, focused, and diligent inquiry); (c) analytic (reasoning, problem resolution, and anticipatory abilities); (d) truth-seeking (pursuit of inquiry, knowledge, and truth); (e) open-minded (divergent views, awareness of self-bias); (f) self-confident (trust in own reasoning); and (g) mature (judicious in decision-making) (Facione, Facione, & Sanchez, 1994, pp. 345-50). To help learners to acquire a critical thinking spirit, faculty must take the initiative to create an open system of learning that fosters such attributes of critical thinking as those cited in the CCTDI.

Cooperative Learning

Educators create the contextual climate of the course that determines the degree and extent of learner involvement. Bevis strongly advocates an educative-caring paradigm which facilitates teacher-student learning-focused interactions and is directed toward achievement of such goals as critical thinking, strategizing, and methods of inquiry (Bevis & Watson, 1989, p. 123). In general, there is a positive correlation between engagement and learning. The more active the learner, the greater the engagement which in turn leads to greater learning (Bevis & Watson, 1989). Consequently, educators must create strategies for student involvement.

Use of small groups for cooperative learning provides a structure that gives students opportunities to actively construct knowledge and develop their cognitive, communication, and decision-making skills. Cooperative learning promotes greater use of higher level reasoning strategies and critical thinking produces more innovative ideas and solutions, and results in a greater transfer of knowledge than individualistic or competitive learning (Johnson, Johnson, & Smith, 1991, p. 2:12). In addition, cooperative learning activities tend to foster positive attitudes toward the content area and the educational experience while increasing motivation for acquiring more knowledge about the subject (Johnson et al., 1991, p. 2:15). Cooperative learning has been found to promote participant achievement, develop higher cognitive abilities, improve communication and problem solving skills, facilitate social interdependence, promote self-esteem, and increase comprehension (McEnerney, 1993, pp. 58-62).

Cooperative learning, a dynamic interactive group process, functions as an open system in which group participants are influenced by all aspects of the environment: the internal, the external, and the created environment as described by Neuman (1995, p. 31). A cooperative milieu should permeate the classroom for at least 60% of the student's learning experiences, whereas up to 40% of the educational processes could be more individualistic and competitive in nature (Johnson et al., 1991, p. 10:9).

Many types of learning are cited as cooperative. However, Johnson et al. (1991), who were instrumental in forming the Cooperative Learning Center at the University of Minnesota, define cooperative learning as the "instructional use of small groups so that students work together to maximize their own and each other's learning" (pp. 1:14 -1:16). In addition, these authors identified five essential elements that differentiate cooperative learning from traditional learning. These elements include: (a) positive group interdependence, (b) face-to-face interaction, (c) individual accountability and personal responsibility, (d) interpersonal and small group skills, and (e) group processing (Johnson et al., 1991, pp. 3:4-3:12).

Teaching and Learning Strategies

The teacher sets the stage for learning. The teacher determines the level of active involvement of students, strategies for teaching, and the structure of learning experiences. Teaching strategies to enhance cognitive development and critical thinking are included in the first clinical course and include the following:

• Encourage students to develop a spirit of inquiry and to be active learners. Establish student relationships through use of inquiry to assist students to discover knowledge within themselves or through group participation. As indicated in the following example, opportunities are readily available for incorporating inquiry and self-discovery into learning situations.

When beginning nursing students are learning basic nursing techniques, they work in groups to practice in a simulated laboratory experience. As two students perform their assigned demonstrations, such as positioning a classmate (client), other students in the clinical group are assigned to critique the procedure. The students who critique are often reluctant to give feedback. They may look quizzically at the faculty member and ask such questions as, "Shouldn't the head of the bed be elevated more?" or "Does he need to have a pillow under his left leg for support?" The faculty member tactfully guides the focus back to the group. The educator may do this by prompting questions to help the students analyze the situation and determine what actions should be taken to position the client properly.

The faculty member may not intercede immediately when students make an error. For instance, if a student demonstrates ambulation while holding a cane in the hand of the simulated affected side, the teacher may ask students if they have any suggestions and then proceed to use inquiry to help students recognize why the action is inappropriate. As students become actively involved in the process, they readily develop working relationships with their peers and tend to respond favorably to constructive criticism in this nonthreatening environment.

• Help students visualize themselves in their role as a nurse and to identify and anticipate events. Require students to contextualize knowledge to various practice settings. Ask questions such as, "As the nurse for Mr. Jones, what would you do if...? How would the nursing care differ for a client with...? How would you teach Mr. Jones to take care of his wound at home?"

• Tell stories that will help students relate to various circumstances, and encourage them to tell stories about their experiences. Telling stories and discussing pertinent aspects of actual situations in the clinical setting provide mental exercises for students to apply theory to practice. For instance, relating your experience about caring for a dying client assists students to gain insight into how to deal with real life events. It also gives students an opportunity to ask such questions as, "What did you say to his wife when he died?"

- Help students learn strategies that will activate memory resources. Help students identify relationships, apply knowledge, and associate material with previous experiences. For instance, sensory memory is acquired through the senses and must be processed quickly to working memory or it will be lost (Carnevali & Thomas, 1993, p. 15). Learning to differentiate which stimuli are significant and require further attention may be especially difficult for the student in a new learning experience. "Did you notice his feet?" may give the student a cue that will prompt recognition of edema which, upon further discussion, may be associated to the condition of congestive heart failure.

- Assist students to use recoding and "chunking" to facilitate the acquisition and retention of information. Memory has a limited capacity of five to nine "chunks"—pieces of mental data. A chunk may contain only one item of information or many related items. Thus, the critical factor for maximizing this aspect of working memory is the size of the chunk. Recoding occurs when related items are grouped together and then remembered as one item (Carnevali & Thomas, 1993, p. 21). For instance, a beginning nursing student may chunk the pulse rate as one item; whereas an experienced nurse may have a cardiac status chunk of data that includes such items as rate, volume, rhythm, activity prior to assessment, skin color, medications, and medical diagnosis. Educators can help students expand their memory by helping them make associations relevant to specific situations. Teachers can also assess the level of learners and build upon students' unique repertoire of knowledge and experiences that influence and shape educational development.

- Other teaching and learning strategies include the use of reframing to stimulate viewing situations from different perspectives, taking initiative to nurture student-teacher interactions, and being present to the student. If a student said that administering a nasogastric feeding was a sterile procedure, the teacher may ask, "If food were administered through the normal oral route, would it be a sterile procedure?"

Newspaper items are also an excellent resource for presenting material from other perspectives. A newspaper column which addresses health care issues cited a letter from a man who had an elevated temperature several days after surgery. He said that he was informed that he had a "staff" infection. He wrote to ask the columnist how one acquires a "staff" infection (Donohue, 1991). What an excellent resource for teaching students about *staph* infections and about staff's involvement in infection control!

- Encourage students to practice professional behaviors, be self-directed, practice assertive behaviors, recognize and reinforce their own achievements, make their learning needs known to appropriate people, and seek assistance when needed. During a project to promote team building, nursing students approached the faculty member and asked her to "talk with staff" about several things that staff could do to improve student-staff interactions. In this situation, students failed to recognize their responsibility to initiate effective communication with staff, to relate their learning needs to staff, and to practice assertive behaviors in assuming their role as a registered nurse student. In response to students' requests and to help resolve a problem that existed between nursing staff and students, team building strategies were implemented. In addition, actions were taken to encourage students to practice assertive behaviors of professional nurses (Freiburger, 1996).

Neuman Systems Model

The Neuman Systems Model provides a comprehensive framework for integrating the course content. The acquisition and application of that content is greatly enhanced by the faculty's use of a wide variety of teaching-learning techniques and strategies in their classes. The ultimate goal of a unique teaching strategy is to promote critical thinking that facilitates the students' abilities to construct and contextualize knowledge in various clinical situations. For example, students, faculty, and clients can be perceived as wholistic beings comprised of Neuman's five variables. In the educational setting, students are taught to draw from resources within the self (knowledge, experiences, observations, thinking abilities) in the realm of the five variables, to think critically, and to make decisions. Application of the students' intellectual abilities is not done in isolation. Context is a significant feature of the process. Nurses use internalized critical thinking skills in conjunction with the interpersonal and extrapersonal environmental forces for cognitive processing and decision making (Neuman, 1995, pp. 10-32). The union of Neuman content with educative-interpretive strategies results in professional nursing education. Subsequent chapters in Unit II will provide specific examples of teaching strategies used in Neuman-based curricula at associate, baccalaureate, and master's levels.

References

American Association of Colleges of Nursing. (1993). **Nursing education's agenda for the 21st century**. Washington, DC: AACN.

Bevis, E.O., & Watson, J. (1989). **Toward a caring curriculum: A new pedagogy for nursing**. New York: National League for Nursing.

Carnevali, D.L., & Thomas, M.D. (1993). **Diagnostic reasoning and treatment decision making in nursing**. Philadelphia: Lippincott.

Donohue, P. (1991, August 27). Staph germs surround us. **The Fort Wayne Journal Gazette**.

Facione, N.C., Facione, P.A., & Sanchez, C.A. (1994). Critical thinking disposition as a measure of competent clinical judgment: The development of the California Critical Thinking Disposition Inventory. **Journal of Nursing Education, 33(8)**, 345-350.

Freiburger, O.A. (1996, November/December). A collaborative approach to team building between students and staff in long term care. **Nurse Educator, 21(6)**, 7-12.

Johnson, D.W., Johnson, R.T., & Smith, K.A. (1991). **Active learning: Cooperation in the college classroom**. Edina, MN: Interaction Book Company.

McEnerney, K. (1993, October). Cooperative learning as a teaching strategy. **Medical Laboratory Observer**, 58-62.

Neuman, B. (1995). **The Neuman Systems Model** (3rd ed.). Norwalk CT: Appleton & Lange.

National League for Nursing. (1990). **Accreditation standards for baccalaureate degree programs and master's degree programs**. New York: Author.

North Central Association of Colleges and Schools. (1992). **A handbook of accreditation**. Chicago: Author.

Paul, R. (1993). Infusing critical thinking into college and university instruction, defining critical thinking. Paper presented at the 1993 critical thinking inservice, Rohnert Park, CA.

Chapter 3
Evaluation in Nursing:
History, Models, and Neuman's Framework
Grace G. Newsome and Lois W. Lowry

Evaluation may be expressed in simple situations as the internal satisfaction of knowing a job has been well done, or it may have widespsread implications such as the granting or removal of an institution's accreditation status. We all continuously participate in evaluation as we informally consider other people's behaviors and activities and as we measure performance formally using established criteria. Within the current environment of managed care and outcomes assessment, evaluation is becoming more detailed and precise for both nursing practice and education.

The purpose of this chapter is to provide a broad overview of the history of evaluation in education and to provide a wholistic definition of evaluation for the educational context. Theorists and models of educational evaluation will be briefly presented and their applicability in Neuman-based programs discussed. Evaluation designs and the importance of outcomes assessment to nursing programs will conclude the chapter.

What is evaluation?

Bevis and Watson (1989, p. 263) provide a definition which states, "Evaluation is a tool; a means for determining merit or worth; a means for providing data or information; and a way to find clues and cues about progress, directions, performance, effectiveness, efficiency, achievement, or usefulness." Effective evaluation is also responsive to the needs, concerns, and perceptions of stakeholders, those with a vested interest in the outcomes of evaluation (Guba & Lincoln, 1989; Scriven, 1980; Stake, 1983). Evaluation must be comprehensive enough in scope and depth to meet the needs of the entity being evaluated, i.e., leading to the demonstration of fulfillment of criteria and rules which are required for accreditation or for approval by agencies such as state boards of nursing. As such, evaluation is wholistic, taking into account the system's environment as well as its parts, processes, and outcomes. Finally, evaluation should result in empowerment to those being evaluated (Guba & Lincoln, 1989).

Educational program evaluation, then, is the collection of information in order to make decisions about the program (Bower, Linc, & Denega, 1988). It encompasses all internal and external forces that influence the program (Welch, Carmody, Murray, & Rafinsky, 1980). Educational program evaluation includes the evaluation of the curriculum, all processes of teaching and learning and their effects on students, work settings, and the community. Data are collected from the school and its students (Dunn, Stockhausen, Thornton, & Barnard, 1995; Jenkins, 1986; Krichbaum, 1994; Oechsle, Volden, & Lambeth, 1990; Ziv, Ehrenfeld, & Hadani, 1990); alumni (Knowles et al.,

1985); employers (Howard, Hubelbank, & Moore, 1989; Ryan & Hodson, 1992); and faculty (Hulsmeyer & Bowling, 1986; Stewart & Hluchyj, 1987).

Historical Aspects of Evaluation

The history of program evaluation in education extends into the 18th century. Madaus, Scriven, and Stufflebeam (1983) outlined six significant periods beginning with the age of reform in the late 18th and 19th centuries. During this period teachers' salaries were determined by how well their students performed in basic reading, spelling, and math. The Boston school system was the first to use test scores as a means of evaluating a school. It is said that Horace Mann used these same test scores as a means to dismiss headmasters who favored corporal punishment (Madaus et al., 1983). In the late 1800s, the first regional accreditation group named the North Central Association of Colleges and Secondary Schools was established. It was not until the 1930s that six additional accrediting bodies were established.

The age of efficiency and testing (1890-1930) emphasized systemization, standardization, and efficiency. Objective-referenced and norm-referenced testing were developed, and evaluation research centered on the local school systems. The use of standardized achievement tests became popular after World War I with the results used to determine program effectiveness. A commercial market arose for achievement tests, especially for school districts that were not large enough to generate their own. Unfortunately, many locally-oriented tests were used to make generalizations about other schools within the state and even the nation.

The Tylerian Age (1930-1945) introduced the idea that test results were not enough unless we knew the test had assessed the meeting of valued objectives. Tyler, known as the father of educational evaluation, conducted the famous "Eight Year Study" in which he looked at the differential effectiveness of various types of schooling. Funded by the Carnegie Corporation, the Eight Year Study compared traditional approaches to education with schools involved in the Progressive Education Movement. Tyler's work in the study resulted in a general rationale for curriculum development and was published as *Basic Principles of Curriculum and Instruction* (Tyler, 1983).

The Age of Innocence (1946-1957) was a postwar period during which many schools were erected. Enrollments in teacher education programs increased dramatically and educational offerings, personnel, and facilities expanded. Following World War II and the depression, America focused on acquiring resources and enjoying a time of peace and prosperity. Little effort or interest was given to holding educators accountable. An increase in standardized testing and increased proficiency in writing objectives was observed. Bloom's Taxonomy was developed to assist educators to write objectives. In 1947, Lindquist, Tyler, and others established the Educational Testing Service (Madaus et al., 1983). Evaluation was still carried out at the local level with the help of local tax money, foundations, and voluntary associations.

The Age of Expansion (1958-1972) saw the passage of the National Defense Education Act. Millions of dollars were put into educational programs, and with the money came a need for concomitant accountability. In 1964 Congress amended the Elementary and Secondary Education Act to include specific evaluation requirements. As a result, Title I under that act required school districts receiving funds to evaluate their work annually. Evaluations of the projects, however, were consistently problematic and almost always yielded negative results. Cronbach cited the lack of relevance and utility of the evaluations as major factors in their results. He advised evaluators to turn away from post hoc experimental methodology that basically compared schools, to more relevant processes such as the reporting of individual test-item scores, that would help guide curriculum development (Madaus et al., 1983).

Difficulty in obtaining satisfactory evaluation data led to the establishment of the National Study Committee on Evaluation. The problem also led to the development of new model conceptualizations by Provus, Eisner, Popham, Cook, Scriven, Stufflebeam, and Stake as they responded to the need to move from a pure Tylerian approach to a more wholistic one that would include the environment, stakeholders, local needs, faculty qualifications, multiple evaluation methodologies, and desired outcome identification (Madaus et al., 1983).

The current Age of Professionalism has seen the evolution of evaluation into a distinct profession (Madaus et al., 1983). Journals, courses, and programs on the subject have been initiated (Berk & Rossi, 1990). In 1980 a Joint Committee appointed by 12 educational evaluation organizations issued a document entitled *Standards for Evaluations of Educational Programs, Projects, and Materials*. These standards were subdivided according to four attributes believed to be critical for any evaluation: utility, feasibility, propriety, and accuracy (Patton, 1988). Scriven (1991) calls this the coming together of a "transdiscipline"— a merging of the tool-disciplines of logic, design, and statistics.

Evaluation Models and Theorists

As the concept of evaluation has matured into a professional discipline, evaluation models have also evolved (Sarnecky, 1990a). This evolution began with models which focused on measurement, such as achievement tests, as the single activity of evaluation. As the need to look at patterns, strengths, and weaknesses became apparent, descriptive models were developed of which Tyler's (1983) model is predominant. Judgment models, such as the work of Scriven, Stake, and Stufflebeam, emerged as the evaluator's role incorporated decision making about the value and worth of the evaluated. The accreditation model for evaluation would also be considered a judgment-focused model.

The current focus is on models which are more qualitative and responsive in nature; they forfeit some quantitative measurement precision to capitalize on the usefulness of the evaluation to the stakeholders. Lincoln and Guba (1985) hold this view and call the approach "responsive evaluation." Responsive evaluation is conducted continuously and interactively with many of the conclusions based on the subjective beliefs of the participants (Guba & Lincoln, 1989; Sarnecky, 1990b). Lincoln and Guba (1985) equate responsive evaluation with a predominantly naturalistic approach that addresses a collaborative relationship with stakeholders, both internal and external.

Another contemporary approach to evaluation is Eisner's (1983) connoisseurship and criticism model. Eisner believes educational evaluators should be the educational equivalent of an art critic. They should view teaching as an art form and schools as cultural phenomena.

Nurses have drawn from models developed in education and other arenas. Tyler's objective-based model has been the most widely used. Waltz (1989a, 1989b), a contemporary nurse evaluator, approaches evaluation of a nursing education program using an eclectic approach that incorporates various other models. The major divisions of her approach include input, processes, and outcomes.

Evaluation models characterize their creators' view of the main concepts involved in evaluation work and provide guidelines for using those concepts to arrive at defensible descriptions, judgments, and recommendations. As such they are "model" views of how to sort and address problems encountered in conducting evaluations (Madaus et al., 1983). Patton (1988) states that few developers of models use their models in pure form. Rather, they approach each evaluation as a problem to be solved and adapt the design of the evaluation to suit the needs of that setting. Patton goes on to say that, "It is perhaps most useful to think of the models, not as either recipes or ideals, but as ideas" (p. 41).

Use of evaluation models enhances the organization and comprehensiveness of the process of evaluation. Selection of a model for nursing program evaluation should be based on the program's philosophy or the nursing theory from which the conceptual framework is developed. Other considerations of selection include the program's resources, personnel time, and priorities established by key interest groups.

In a study by Brady and Netusil (1988), it was found that program evaluation plans were used in 94% of nursing education programs surveyed. However, only 43% of the schools were using one particular evaluation model; 80% of respondents stated that an evaluation model would be helpful. The models reported in use include Stufflebeam's context, input, process, and product (CIPP) model (Bevil, 1991; Clark, Goodwin, Mariani, Marshall, & Moore, 1983), Guba and Lincoln's responsive model (Meyers, 1990; Sarnecky, 1990b), and Provus' discrepancy model (Stewart & Hluchyj, 1987).

The most common models used in education are described in the following paragraphs and in **Table 3.1**.

Table 3.1: Evaluation Models

Model/Author	Major Focus/Purpose	Methodology
Objective based/ Tyler	Use of objectives	Quantitative
	To measure and describe student progress/ outcomes in relation to stated objectives.	Formative and summative measurement of objectives
CIPP/ Stufflebeam	Decision making	Questionnaire and interview surveys
	Context, input, process, and product evaluation guides planning, structuring, implementation, and recycling decisions.	
Goal Free/ Scriven	Valuing	Comparative summative evaluation
	Decision making	
	Reduces bias with measurement of all outcomes, intended and unintended.	Use of key evaluation checklist
Countenance/ Stake	Responsive evaluation Emphasis on describing and judging the program, not the educational product.	Case study Qualitative
	Description and judgement of antecedents, transactions, and outcomes.	
Educational critic/ Eisner	Educational connoisseurship and criticism	Primarily qualitative
	To evaluate education within context of teaching as an art form and schooling as a cultural phenomenon; judgement of educational value by one who is a connoisseur of education.	
Naturalistic inquiry/ Guba	Grounded theory Contextual relevance	Qualitative study Natural setting Case-study format
Accreditation	Peer evaluation to determine program quality.	Self-study; site visits
	Granting of approval or accreditation by professional organization.	Measurement of criteria against standards
		Primarily quantitative
Waltz	Determines the Who, Why, What, When, How, and Major Audience of evaluation.	Quantitative and qualitative
	Consideration of inputs, processes, and outcomes.	

Tyler's Model. Tyler's (1983) objective-based model originated in the 1940s, ahead of its time in comparison to other frequently-used models. The use of this model moved evaluation from the sole use of test scores to a broader more inclusive approach. No longer were measurements taken simply to have scores which reflected the ability of individual students. Rather, the measurement of specific objectives was done to determine if the objectives were being met (Waltz, 1989a). This included reviewing objectives in relation to student characteristics, content to be learned, and type of learning desired. Tyler brought a sweeping change to educational evaluation, a change which still has a major influence on how education is conducted. Indeed, this model has been the most widely used of all models of evaluation (Stufflebeam & Webster, 1983).

As a descriptive model, its methodology is rooted in positivist or quantitative approaches. Nursing education found the specific delineation of cognitive and affective objectives as well as the determination of congruence between objectives and learning experiences extremely useful. Many basic nursing programs continue to make significant use of the model (Waltz, 1989a). The Tylerian model is widely used in the design of clinical evaluation instruments. Cecil Community College, Indiana University-Purdue University at Ft. Wayne, and University of Tennessee provide examples of instruments based on this approach in chapters in Unit III. According to critics, weaknesses of Tyler's model include the fact that it is primarily summative in nature and that it basically ignores the context of the educational process, the external factors, and the stakeholders who affect the program (Waltz, 1989a).

Stufflebeam's CIPP Model. Decision-making is the central theme of Stufflebeam's (1983) approach to educational evaluation. He recommends that evaluators and decision-makers be distinct (separate). The role of evaluators is to collect and present information and alternatives to decision makers who are generally internal to the program being evaluated. Stufflebeam's CIPP model of evaluation incorporates the idea of context as a viable component of evaluation. Considering the context enables stakeholders to guide planning based on their needs, ideas, and values. Input evaluation provides information related to the utilization of resources and includes a cost-benefit perspective (Waltz, 1989a). Process evaluation gives feedback as the program is implemented, and product evaluation measures program outcomes. Results of outcome measurement lead to what Stufflebeam refers to as recycling decisions; that is, decisions on how the program will be revised, supported, or managed that will create better or different outcomes. A major advantage of this type of decision-oriented model is that it encourages the continuous and systematic use of evaluation as programs are planned, implemented, and revised (Waltz, 1989a). Principles from this model are used by nursing programs seeking or maintaining accreditation. An example of the systematic process in use at Lander University is described in Chapter 14.

Stake's Countenance Model. Stake (1983) refers to considering the context as being responsive. This concept of "responding" to the milieu and its constituents is a major component of Stake's countenance or responsive model approach. The model includes describing and judging based on examinations of the antecedent (conditions that existed before program processes), of transaction (succession of engagements that comprise the program process), and of outcome (immediate and long-term effects of a program on participants, clients, and others in the community) phases of the program (Waltz, 1989a). In Stake's model the evaluator finds out what is of value to the audience of clients, professional groups, and program staff and gathers expressions of worth from various people, whose points of view differ. Stake emphasizes letting the evaluation emerge from observing the program. That is, he focuses more on program activities than program intents. Stake (1980) identifies 12 events that occur in responsive evaluation and which are inherently facilitated by an external evaluator. Stake (1978) relies significantly on qualitative methods and frequently uses case study within this context. Several chapters in Unit III illustrate this model.

Scriven's Goal-Free Model. Scriven's (1973) model of evaluation is called Goal-Free Evaluation. The intent of Scriven's model is to have the evaluator "discover" all of the program's effects. A knowledge of the program's specific goals, objectives, or outcomes is not used by the evaluators when conducting the evaluation; they are guided instead by Scriven's Key Evaluation Checklist which is a list of dimensions and questions that illuminate evaluation data. Evaluators match the program's effects against the needs of those that the program is to serve and/or compare them to standards of merit. Goal-free evaluation requires the use of external evaluators to ensure that bias does not effect evaluation results.

Scriven's many contributions to evaluation theory included the introduction of such terms as formative and summative, metaevaluation, and goal-free evaluation. Formative and summative processes are commonly used in nursing education programs. Scriven's "Logic of Valuing" legitimized the fact that evaluation inherently involves values and should explicitly recognize this. He argues that society requires a science of valuing before it will be able to know if its programs are indeed good. Another component of Scriven's multimodel to reduce bias in evaluation is metaevaluation, whereby the evaluation process is also evaluated.

Accreditation Model. Accreditation is the process by which an external organization grants approval to an educational institution. While there is no one person who initiated the accreditation approach, one of the earliest uses of this approach is reflected in Flexner's (1910) Report. Flexner's study of medical education in the United States and Canada ultimately led to the closing of many medical schools of poor quality and the merging of many others for the purposes of sharing resources and improving their outcomes. Since that time, multiple accrediting bodies have been formed in education and function under the guidance of the Council on Postsecondary Accreditation (COPA). The accreditation model uses self-study, site visits, and peer reviewers as its main components. Specific goals of programs are criteria for determining success; objectives are stated in measurable terms. Outcome indicates whether goals were attained. The main advantage of having accreditation is that it helps determine the quality of educational institutions and programs (Stufflebeam & Webster, 1983). The accreditation process is widely accepted by nurse educators who wish endorsement for a high-quality program. Although the National League for Nursing (NLN) is now the accrediting body for nursing, this may change in the future. All the programs cited in this monograph are NLN accredited.

Guba and Lincoln's Naturalistic Model. Lincoln and Guba (1985) report the use of a responsive model using naturalistic inquiry/qualitative methodology. They support this view over the more frequently used quantitative approaches by stating that no one "reality" exists—only realities that we construct. They say that valid knowledge is that which best portrays the rich and individual variations of each person's created reality. They recognize that the inquirer and the object of inquiry are inseparable and that they interact to influence one another (Lincoln & Guba, 1985). These interacting influences make it impossible to establish causal linkages. While other models promote use of qualitative methods, such as Stake's primary use of the case study approach, Lincoln and Guba view the naturalistic approach as more than a method. It is a paradigm that guides all of the evaluator's work. As a constructivist, Guba not only "abjures objectivity," he "celebrates subjectivity" (Guba, 1990, p. 17). The evaluation process at Yakima Community College blends Guba's naturalistic method with responsive evaluation (Stake, 1983) to produce an innovative clinical evaluation process. Further discussion is in Chapter 12.

Eisner's Educational Connoisseurship and Criticism Model. Eisner (1985) has applied his background in art to educational evaluation. He believes that education would be greatly improved if the techniques of art criticism were applied to the evaluation process. He thinks the development of the mind is a cultural achievement and that curriculum and teaching methods are artistic means for creating minds (Eisner, 1990). He deemphasizes the fixed mental capability of any given student and, instead, challenges educators to create learning experiences that will cultivate and "grow the mind." By this, he means implementing curricula which will provide "mind-altering" experiences (Eisner, 1990, p. 90). Incorporating the art critic approach would lead to multiple ways of knowing, a more synergistic, integrated curriculum, and ultimately, a more integrated, wholistically functioning student and graduate. Eisner's model is congruent with the educative-interpretive model. An educator must grapple with the complex task of finding ways to assess "mind altering" growth and learning.

Waltz's Nursing Model. Waltz (1989a, 1989b) views program evaluation as a decision-making process that includes the program's inputs (participant's talents, skills, and aspirations; their cultures, families, and nurse specialties; and money, time, and other resources available); processes (program procedures and techniques; content; styles of those who administer and implement the program; and environmental and psychological contexts within which the program is implemented); and outcomes (results in light of goals and objectives and in relation to the specific information needs of decision-makers). This eclectic approach is summarized by determining the Who, Why, What, When, How, and Major Audience of evaluation (Waltz, 1989a). Specific strategies and techniques for developing and implementing a master plan using Waltz's approach are outlined in Waltz's (1989b) "Evaluating the Program."

Educational Evaluation and Neuman's Framework

Neuman-based educational programs were developed in the 1970s and 1980s and were influenced by the Tylerian (behaviorist) model. Tyler's (1983) emphasis on measurable goals and objectives leads to a prescription of behaviors to be evaluated for the measurement of student learning. Faculty teaching in model-based programs would design tests and use instruments stemming from Neuman concepts that were deemed essential to students learning. Some instruments measured student clinical and classroom competencies, others measured depth and breadth of client care as noted in care plans. Although the Neuman Systems Model presents a broad and comprehensive framework based on theories of wholism, systems, and gestalt, when it is adopted by educators with a behaviorist bias, much of the richness and creativity of the model is at risk of loss as faculty attempt to reduce the model propositions to fit specific objectives. Behaviorist theory supports the learning typologies of item, directive, and rationale learning that are vital to training and skill development for nurses. This typology, however, cannot and does not include the affective domain, valuing, nor critical thinking that is vital to the development of professional behaviors. Evaluation becomes the "driver" in behaviorist curricula. To capture breadth and depth of experiences, an eclectic approach to evaluation must be taken.

The Neuman Systems Model provides philosophical parameters and an organizing structure for the curriculum. The model definitions of person, environment, health, and nursing and the basic assumptions of the model provide a language and perspective that can guide faculty in the design of a consistent plan to guide teaching, student practice, and evaluation throughout the curriculum. However, the reductionism required by behaviorist typology often frustrates faculty, thus limiting the creative potential of the model.

Neuman's world view of organicism, wholism, client-nurse perceptions, and interactions would most appropriately be evaluated through a broader variety of evaluation processes including formative, responsive, and qualitative. Formative evaluation is a teaching opportunity in which teacher and learner collaborate to help students achieve their goals. The teacher in this mode is perceived as an expert learner and co-learner within the educative process and evaluation becomes a growth experience, rather than a test. Unforeseen learnings are as important for student growth as intended ones.

Evaluation becomes a shared teacher-learner activity in which there is reflection on meanings of experiences and patterns of behavior (Bevis and Watson, 1989). Responsive evaluation through qualitative approaches, such as client case studies based on Neuman's preventions as intervention, can provide opportunities for faculty-student exchanges that result in individual variations of each person's created reality. Learning and growth occur.

We have discussed in Chapter One the Neuman Systems Model as an appropriate framework for contextual, syntactical, and inquiry learning; the typologies espoused for professional teaching and learning. Thus, evaluation strategies selected by educators of professional nurses must be consistent with the goals of these typologies—e.g., critical thinking, inquiry, and visualization of new possibilities. Evaluation processes are more difficult when "goals" become all that educators and students have to guide their endeavors. This "looseness" of structure may be disturbing for faculty who are more familiar with the behaviorist model and tend to "reduce the model" to specific objectives for evaluation. This practice tends to contain and restrain rather than to liberate students in their learning. If faculty select a comprehensive nursing model such as Neuman's framework to guide professional curriculum development, they need to use evaluation models that are consistent with the theoretical foundation of the nursing model.

Educators who teach from the educative-interpretive paradigm need to select evaluation models that are naturalistic, wholistic, responsive, and contextual (Eisner, 1985; Guba & Lincoln, 1989; Stake, 1983). These models are guided by the belief that the most meaningful evaluation comes from personal perceptions; thus, these models are sensitive to multiple points of view—especially views of those with a stake in the program. Evaluation data is collected through qualitative methods and naturalistic studies. Such an approach will provide evaluation data that is accurate and rich.

Evaluation Design

The major thrust of evaluation designers has been quantitative. Cook and Campbell (1979) insisted on rigorous experimental designs to assure program effectiveness. Campbell's methodological work on causation forged the strongest links between Campbell and evaluation practice. Others support this experimental approach believing that biases can result from an evaluator's personal observations and intuitive analyses.

Lincoln and Guba (1985) argue that the experimental approach alienates stakeholders who are most affected by the program. Their opinions and concerns are subject to stringent data collection techniques and statistical tests of significance. Guba and Lincoln (1987, 1989) support the use of naturalistic inquiry as a primary mode of evaluation data collection. They hold to the belief that data stem from interactions, for only then can the true intentions of respondents be known. They are postpositivist in their approach, believing this approach has greater success in determining truth than the positivist who employs causal techniques (Lincoln & Guba, 1985). Presented in Chapter 12 is an evaluation design now in use at Yakima Valley Community College (Washington) and based on Guba's fourth-generation work.

Chen (1990) supports the use of both experimental and naturalistic approaches. He believes that what is most important is the use of program theory to illuminate the priority of the foci of evaluation, which will in turn determine the method of evaluation best suited for the program. Chen believes that using program theory will also aid the testing of the theory itself. Weiss (1972) concurs with Chen and attributes the low utilization of evaluation data to the lack of theory driving the evaluation. Cronbach also agrees that evaluation should be a program of studies with a mixture of styles and design, asserting that only in this way is it likely that the "full truth" of the situation will be assessed (Shrinkfield, 1983). Each method of evaluation, quantitative or qualitative, is associated with separate and unique paradigmatic perspectives that are seemingly incongruent. It appears that quantitative methods have been developed most directly for the task of verifying or confirming theories and that to a large extent qualitative methods were purposely developed for the task of discovering or generating theories. While this division is not so clear in nursing there has been a definite shift from the behaviorist mode of thinking to a less prescriptive approach (Bevis, 1989; Whiteley, 1992). The National League for Nursing's publication, *A Vision for Nursing Education* (1993), recognizes the move among nursing scholars from a prevailing paradigm of logical positivism to more qualitative work. This shift must be translated into the practical world of nursing education. Educators are challenged to select evaluation models that will truly elicit the kind of data needed to make program decisions.

Outcome Assessment

Herbener and Watson (1992) define outcomes as the abilities, achievements, attitudes, and aspirations of students that result from the educational experience. Hart and Waltz (1988) define outcomes as the outputs or results of the program or the activities of the provider. According to the National League for Nursing (1990, p. 1), outcomes can be differentiated from the traditional accreditation criteria in that "criteria focus on the capability of the program; they are those factors which enable a faculty to meet their stated goals and objectives." Outcome criteria, on the other hand, "focus on whether or not the program is actually effective in doing what it says it will do and for which it has demonstrated its capability" (p. 1). The evaluation plan of Indiana University Purdue University, Fort Wayne incorporates a comprehensive outcomes assessment for program evaluation and development. This plan is described in detail in Chapter 16.

A major research effort to determine the status of outcome assessment in nursing education was conducted by the National League for Nursing with grant support from the Helene Fuld foundation (Hart & Waltz, 1988; Waltz & Neuman, 1988). The NLN's research indicated that most studies cited in the literature were predictive ones in which student characteristics, course grades, or cumulative grade point averages were analyzed in an effort to predict scores on the state board examination. Student outcomes most often evaluated by the majority of schools were academic achievement, the nursing care plan, and implementation of the plan of care (Waltz, 1988). Only one-half of nursing schools reported measuring outcomes prior to and after graduation and only slightly more than half of the schools indicated that findings were very important in making decisions regarding program quality and effectiveness (Waltz, 1988). Less than one fourth of the schools reported using findings obtained from employees, graduates, and applicants to the program.

A very significant finding was that only two percent of schools in the study reported evaluating outcomes other than student outcomes (Waltz, 1988). According to Waltz it was apparent that more attention must be given to the selection of outcomes deemed important to those outside the organization. Examples might include employer satisfaction with graduates, preparedness of graduates to provide population-based care, and client satisfaction with delivery of care. She also saw as important the need for assessment of affective outcomes such as leadership, critical thinking, and creativity.

These concerns are critically linked to the problems facing nursing, health care, and health care reform. In other words, Waltz believes that nurses' ability to have an effect on the current health care dilemma and transformation depends on a greater focus on multiple outcome assessments and the development of thinking skills that promote independence and autonomy in graduates. Waltz recommends the development and testing of evaluation instruments in this regard (Waltz, 1988).

Chapters 15 and 16 contain evaluation studies of graduates to determine their internalization of Neuman's propositions and their perceptions on how useful Neuman's model has been in their delivery of client care. Neuman's model also emphasizes outcomes of nursing goals and interventions through its nursing process format. Client goal-outcomes validate the nursing process. Educators in Neuman-based programs should use students' client care plans as an evaluation of inquiry learning.

In conclusion, the outcome assessment revolution arose from an educational crisis in our society. State officials have quickly fallen into line to require the assessment of learning outcomes. Nurse educators, through the NLN, incorporated outcomes in the criteria for accreditation required of all programs for the self-study report and NLN accreditation visit. With the current trends in health care and higher education it is expected that outcome assessment, as part of the evaluation process, will increase as accountability to individual consumers and the public plays an ever larger role in the move toward high-quality and cost-efficient, population-based care. Indeed, faculty must incorporate several evaluation models within their programs to truly enhance the merit, value, effectiveness, achievement, and usefulness of their programs of learning.

References

Berk, R.A., & Rossi, P.H. (1990). **Thinking about program evaluation**. Newbury Park: Sage.

Bevil, C.A. (1991). **Program evaluation in nursing education: Creating a meaningful plan.** A presentation at the National League for Nursing convention. Nashville: Author.

Bevis, E.O. (1989). **Curriculum building in nursing.** (3rd ed.) New York: National League for Nursing.

Bevis, E.O., & Watson, J. (1989). **Toward the caring curriculum: A new pedagogy for nursing.** New York: National League for Nursing.

Bower, D., Linc, L., & Denega, D. (1988). **Evaluation instruments in nursing.** New York: National League for Nursing.

Brady, L., & Netusil, A. (1988). A national study of nursing educations' use of a model of program evaluation. **Journal of Nursing Education, 27,** 225-226.

Chen, H. (1990). **Theory-driven evaluations.** Newbury Park: Sage.

Clark, T., Goodwin, M., Mariani, M., Marshall, M.J., & Moore, S. (1983). Curriculum evaluation: An application of Stufflebeam's model in a baccalaureate school of nursing. **Journal of Nursing Education, 22(2),** 54-58.

Cook, T.D., & Campbell, D.T. (1979). **Quasi-experimentation: Design and analysis issues for field settings.** Chicago: Rand McNally.

Dunn, S.V., Stockhausen, L., Thornton, R., & Barnard, A. (1995). The relationship between clinical education format and selected student learning outcomes. **Journal of Nursing Education, 34(1),** 16-24.

Eisner, E.W. (1983). Educational Connoisseurship and Criticism: Their Form and Functions in Educational Evaluation. In G.F. Madaus, M.S. Scriven, & D.L. Stufflebeam (Eds.), **Evaluation models, viewpoints on educational and human service evaluation.** Boston-Kluwer-Nijhoff.

Eisner, E.W. (1985). **The educational imagination: On the design and evaluation of educational programs** (2nd ed.). New York: Macmillan.

Eisner, E.W. (1990). The meaning of alternative paradigms for practice. In E.G. Guba (Ed.), **The paradigm dialog.** Newbury Park: Sage.

Flexner, A. (1910). Medical education in the United States and Canada. Bulletin no. 4. New York: Carnegie Foundation for the Advancement of Teaching.

Guba, E.G. (Ed.). (1990). The paradigm dialog. Newbury Park: Sage.

Guba, E.G., & Lincoln, Y.S. (1987). The countenances of fourth generation evaluation: Description, judgement, and negotiation. In D.J. Palumbo (Ed.), **The politics of program evaluation.** Newbury Park: Sage.

Guba, E.G., & Lincoln, Y.S. (1989). **Fourth generation evaluation.** Newbury Park: Sage.

Hart, S.E., & Waltz, C.F. (1988). **Educational outcomes: Assessment of quality-state of the art and future directions.** New York: National League for Nursing.

Herbener, D.J., & Watson, J.E. (1992). Models for evaluating nursing education programs. **Journal of Nursing Education, 40(1),** 27-32.

Howard, E., Hubelbank, J., & Moore, P. (1989). Employer evaluation of graduates: Use of the focus group. **Nurse Educator, 14(5),** 38-41.

Hulsmeyer, B.S., & Bowling, A.K. (1986). Evaluating colleagues' classroom teaching effectiveness. **Nurse Educator, 11(5),** 19-23.

Jenkins, H.M. (1986). Student participation in curriculum evaluation. **Nurse Educator, 11(5),** 16-18.

Knowles, L.N., Strozier, V.R., Wilson, J.M., Bodo, T.L., Greene, D.B., & Sarver, V.T. (1985). Evaluation of a baccalaureate nursing program by alumni and of alumni by their supervisors. **Journal of Nursing Education, 24(6),** 261-264.

Krichbaum, K. (1994). Clinical teaching effectiveness described in relation to learning outcomes of baccalaureate nursing students. **Journal of Nursing Education, 33(7),** 306-315.

Lincoln, Y.S., & Guba, E.G. (1985). **Naturalistic inquiry.** Newberry Park: Sage.

Madaus, G.F., Scriven, M.S., & Stufflebeam, D.L. (Eds.) (1983). **Evaluation models, viewpoints on educational and human service evaluation.** Boston: Kluwer-Nijhoff.

Meyers, S.K. (1990). Program evaluation for accreditation. **American Journal of Occupational Therapy, 44(9),** 823-826.

National League for Nursing. (1990). Some of the Most Commonly Asked Questions About Outcomes. New York: NLN Division of Education and Accreditation, November.

National League for Nursing. (1993). A Vision for Nursing Education. New York: National League for Nursing, Publication # 14-2581.

Oechsle, L., Volden, S.L., & Lambeth, M. (1990). Portfolios and RNs: An evaluation. **Journal of Nursing Education, 29(2)**, 54-59.

Patton, M.Q. (1988). **Practical evaluation**. Newbury Park: Sage.

Ryan, M.E., & Hodson, K.E. (1992). Employer evaluations of nurse graduates: A critical program assessment element. **Journal of Nursing Education, 31(5)**, 198-202.

Sarnecky, M. (1990a). Program evaluation. Part I: Four generations of theory. **Nurse Educator, 15(5)**, 25-28.

Sarnecky, M. (1990b). Program evaluation. Part 2: A responsive model proposal. **Nurse Educator, 15(6)**, 7-10.

Scriven, M. (1973). Goal-free evaluation. In E.R. House (Ed.), **School evaluation: The politics and process**. Berkeley, CA: McCutchan.

Scriven, M. (1980). **The logic of evaluation**. Inverness, CA: Edgepress.

Scriven, M. (1991). **Evaluation thesaurus** (4th ed.). Newbury Park: Sage.

Shrinkfield, A.J. (1983). Designs for evaluations of educational and social progress by Lee J. Cronvich: A synopsis. In G.F. Madaus, M.S. Scriven, & D.L. Stufflebeam (Eds.), **Evaluation models, viewpoints on educational and human service evaluation**. Boston: Kluwer-Nijhoff.

Stake, R.E. (1978). The case study method in social inquiry. **Educational Researcher, 7**, 5-8.

Stake, R.E. (1980). Program evaluation, particularly responsive evaluation. In W.B. Dockrell & D. Hamilton (Eds.), **Rethinking educational research**. London: Hodder & Stoughton.

Stake, R. E. (1983). Program evaluation, particularly responsive evaluation. In G.F. Madaus, M.S. Scriven, & D.L. Stufflebeam (Eds.), **Evaluation models, viewpoints on educational and human service evaluation**. Boston: Kluwer-Nijhoff.

Stewart, J., & Hluchyj, T. (1987). An approach to nursing curriculum evaluation. **Nursing Outlook, 35(2)**, 79-81.

Stufflebeam, D.L. (1983). The CIPP model of program evaluation. In G.F. Madaus, M.S. Scriven, & D.L. Stufflebeam (Eds.), **Evaluation models, viewpoints on educational and human service evaluation**. Boston: Kluwer-Nijhoff.

Stufflebeam, D.L., & Webster, W.J. (1983). An analysis of alternative approaches to evaluation. In G.F. Madaus, M.S. Scriven, & D.L. Stufflebeam (Eds.), **Evaluation models, viewpoints on educational and human service evaluation**. Boston: Kluwer-Nijhoff

Tyler, R.W. (1983). A rationale for program evaluation. In G.F. Madaus, M.S. Scriven, & D.L. Stufflebeam (Eds.), **Evaluation models, viewpoints on educational and human service evaluation**. Boston: Kluwer-Nijhoff

Waltz, C.F. (1988). Survey of schools. In S.E. Hart & C.F. Waltz (Eds.), **Educational outcomes: Assessment of quality—state of the art and future directions**. New York: National League for Nursing.

Waltz, C.F. (1989a). Program evaluation. In C.F. Waltz, S.B. Chambers, & N.B. Hechenberger (Eds.), **Strategic planning, marketing, and evaluation for nursing education and service**. New York: National League for Nursing.

Waltz, C.F., (1989b). Evaluating the program. In C.F. Waltz, S.B. Chambers, & N.B. Hechenberger (Eds.), **Strategic planning, marketing, and evaluation for nursing education and service**. New York: National League for Nursing.

Waltz, C.F., & Neuman, L.H. (1988). (Eds.). **Educational outcomes: assessment of quality—compendium of measurement tools for associate degree nursing programs**. New York: National League for Nursing.

Welch, L.B., Carmody, C., Murray, M., & Rafinsky, L. (1980). Program evaluation: An overview. **Nursing and Health Care, 1(4)**, 186-191.

Weiss, C.H. (1972). **Evaluation research: Methods for assessing program effectiveness**. Englewood Cliffs, NJ: Prentice-Hall.

Whiteley, S. (1992). Evaluation of nursing education programmes—theory and practice. **International Journal of Nursing Studies, 29(3)**, 315-323.

Ziv, L., Ehrenfeld, M., & Hadani, P.E. (1990). Student evaluation of the school program. **Journal of Nursing Education, 29(2)**, 60-65.

Unit II: Strategies for the Journey

"Tell me and I may remember.
Show me and I understand."
—Chinese Proverb

Education for the future involves interactive processes among students, faculty, and clients that demonstrate caring and commitment to self and others. Theory and practice inform each other in praxis. Chapters in Unit II present innovative teaching-learning strategies that infuse critical thinking, caring, and cooperative learning within Neuman-based curricula.

Chapter 4
Critical Thinking, the Neuman Systems Model, and Associate Degree Education

Sarah J. Beckman, Sanna Boxley-Harges,
Cheryl Bruick-Sorge, and Judith Eichenauer

Nurse educators are challenged to develop, nurture, and evaluate critical thinking skills in nursing students. These skills are essential to sound clinical judgments in practice settings. Critical thinking skills are learned in classroom environments that are dynamic, decentralized, and interactive (Jerit & Taylor, 1992). Nursing models can provide the framework for the leveling of nursing content while creative teaching strategies provide the process by which students learn to develop critical thinking.

The Indiana University-Purdue University at Fort Wayne (IPFW) associate degree nursing program integrates the Neuman Systems Model throughout the curriculum, thus providing a framework within which students learn to make clinical decisions. When the Department of Nursing adopted the Betty Neuman Systems Model in the associate degree program in 1982, Dr. Neuman assisted the faculty with implementation. Teaching materials were then developed that continue to be revised and used today. Teaching/learning strategies that promote critical thinking and faculty-student interaction are consistently used throughout the curriculum.

The educational process at IPFW is based on several theories. Kurt Lewin's principles of change, decision making, unfreezing, moving, and refreezing (Lewin, 1951) undergird the process. The nursing process provides the decision-making model for case scenarios analyzed in the classroom as well as for client situations encountered in the clinical setting. The Neuman Systems Model guides and directs decision making at each stage of the nursing process. The first four levels of Bloom's taxonomy are used to direct teaching activities and content and in assessing student performance (Anderson & Sosniak, 1994).

Strategies that encourage critical thinking are: presenting case scenarios, encouraging active participation, using demonstration/role modeling followed by small group analysis and discussion, thinking aloud with the faculty member in preparation for the presentation, and collaborative learning activities with peers. An important consideration in developing critical thinking by students is acknowledgment of human imperfection and identification of "room for error." There is more room for error when thinking aloud and discussing with faculty than when actually caring for a client. Providing a risk-free environment in which mistakes can be made while learning, discussing, and thinking is emphasized. Faculty seek to create the least threatening environment for productive learning. Strategies used in specific courses are discussed in this chapter.

Level-One Courses

The Neuman Systems Model is introduced to students in the first nursing course, NUR 115, "Nursing of the Adult." The model is presented through the use of slides and a transparency with overlays that can depict the individual components of the schematic diagram of the model. Each component is defined and examples are cited to further aid understanding.

One creative teaching initiative that imprints the model on the minds of associate degree students occurs when baccalaureate students present the Neuman Model via a videotaped presentation. In this video, five students interpret the Neuman Model and illustrate the major concepts through a case scenario. Each RN-BS student actor portrays one component part of the model; together the actors form circles to depict the central core, lines of resistance, and lines of defense. The RN-BS students "think aloud" while using the model to analyze a case scenario. The case scenario depicts a nursing student as client who is enrolled for 18 credit hours and whose financial aid did not get approved. The student is diagnosed with mononucleosis with the symptoms of insomnia, poor eating habits, and a lack of regular aerobic exercise. As the situation worsens, the student client is hospitalized. Following the video, discussion about the model is facilitated by the faculty member. Student feedback indicates that the role play is a helpful tool in assisting them to understand model concepts.

In the fourth week of the 15-week semester, the nursing process is introduced along with the Department of Nursing Assessment Guide and Nursing Process Tool. The guide and tool are organized according to the total person approach (Neuman, 1995) that incorporates the five client variables and the concepts of personal stressors. In the clinical setting students assess clients according to the items listed on the guide, identify nursing diagnoses from the assessment data they have gathered, and write a care plan for each diagnosis. Criteria established for the grading of the care plans require that the paper demonstrate interpretation and analysis of data as well as synthesis of knowledge. For example, one criterion requires that the student define the chronic health conditions and relate them to the current health status of the client. Further, the student must include diagnostic test data and correlate the results to the client's condition. This criterion requires critical thinking skills such as in-depth analysis, logical reasoning, and making appropriate decisions. Student knowledge is truly demonstrated through their care plans.

In the second 100-level course, NUR 116, "Nursing of the Adult II," the Nursing Diagnosis Guide is introduced to assist students to analyze and synthesize assessment data before the actual writing of the nursing care plan. The link between the Nursing Assessment Guide and the Nursing Process Tool is used to guide students through the thinking processes. The Nursing Diagnosis Guide tool is composed of four parts. In part one, as problems are derived from the cue clusters, three lists of stressors are developed: intra-, inter-, and extrapersonal.

Part two continues thought process development by directing students to draw arrows for each identified stressor into the NSM circular diagram of flexible and normal lines of defense, lines of resistance, and core structure. For each stressor the degree of arrow penetration varies. The student is required to write a brief explanation identifying the reason for the selected degree of penetration of each arrow. For example, the students need to explain why a stressor whose arrow penetrates through all lines of defense is life threatening while arrows that only penetrate the flexible line of defense are not life threatening.

In part three, students explore how the client's flexible line of defense can be strengthened or maintained through teaching and health/wellness promotion. This activity promotes continuity in nursing care-plan development and helps students consider client strengths, both in the development of the care plan and in selection of therapeutic nursing interventions. Finally, students prioritize and write nursing diagnoses which are based on Neuman concepts and principles.

Level-Two Courses

In 200-level nursing courses, strategies employed in previous courses continue to be used as others are added. The use of case scenarios brings to life the content in Nursing of the Adult III, through clients who have real problems and needs. Frequently, these scenarios are real events that have been experienced by students in the clinical setting. Faculty begin by giving a brief content presentation followed by a case scenario. The faculty member "thinks aloud" and models critical thinking as the Neuman Model is used to analyze the data. Students are selected or may volunteer to identify stressors—intra-, inter-, extra-personal for this client. Students identify the depth to which each stressor penetrates the lines of defense. Students then select areas in which the client's flexible line of defense can be strengthened or maintained, providing implications for teaching and health promotion (tertiary preventions). Students formulate nursing diagnoses prioritized according to Maslow's hierarchy of needs. Faculty and students discuss all interventions—primary, secondary, and tertiary—for each diagnosis.

Critical thinking skills are improved through analysis of case scenarios, group discussion, and collaborative learning. Learning occurs as students receive immediate and/or corrective feedback and experience room for error. Prior learning is reinforced through application of the nursing process and discipline-specific knowledge. New content is presented through case scenarios. Student feedback to the faculty about this strategy has included comments such as, "Case studies really put it all together;" "I really feel I learn from case scenarios because it makes me think in class;" and "I remember material much more easily after the case scenario is discussed in class."

It is vital that students are able to transfer knowledge from class to clinical applications. At this point "risk" has increased and the "room for error" has lessened dramatically. Faculty in the clinical setting must be skilled strategists employing teaching strategies that are timely, stimulating to critical thinking, and appropriate to the situation. Conference time is utilized to its maximum potential.

A postconference strategy that promotes critical thinking is a group case study analysis. Students are divided into groups of two or three. Each group is given a written client case which is "typical" of clients cared for in the practicum setting who may have special needs related to ethical considerations or discharge planning. Ten minutes is allowed for case discussion. One student is the recorder. Other students collaboratively analyze the situation and determine the severity of stressor penetration, formulate a prioritized problem list or nursing diagnoses, and list major nursing interventions for each nursing diagnosis. The NSM is the organizing framework for providing wholistic client care. After the allotted time, students present their case to the entire class. Feedback by peers and faculty leads to lively and informative interaction. Students evaluate this strategy positively and value the opportunity to apply previous learning. They also indicate that the feedback they receive from other students is a positive experience. Faculty use this strategy to assess group interaction as well as the ability of students to transfer knowledge to the practice setting.

Other clinical strategies include the "Nursing Care Project," oral presentation, and individual mentoring. The "Nursing Care Project," a 30-45 minute oral report on an assigned client, is a strategy used in pre/postconference. The choice of the patient is mutually decided upon by the student and faculty member. Preparation before the clinical activity of the project includes reading, review of theory content, critically thinking about the needs, stressors, and care of clients, and formulating questions that are unanswered in the manual or which require clarification. Students are required to delay patient selection until they have cared for several patients so that they have gained adequate experience. This is difficult for some students as they are anxious "to get started." According to Lewin's principles, decision making and unfreezing has begun, resulting in change within cognitive, psychomotor, and affective knowledge or skills.

In preparation for the project, the faculty member identifies clients who have multiple stressors and require secondary as well as tertiary and primary interventions. The learning plan for each student is individualized based on his/her current knowledge and skill level. The goal is to reasonably challenge the student to apply previous learning to new scenarios and/or to learn new information, disease processes, and psychomotor skills. When students apply previous learning to new situations, they experience increased self confidence.

Many students are uncomfortable presenting material to a group. One creative teaching strategy which eases some of this tension and reassures students is to have students give a 3-5 minute "mini presentation." Approved topics include skills learned and experienced in the 100-level courses, such as "SQ/IM" injection sites, types and care of nasogastric tubes, and pain management. Anticipated patient stressors related to these topics are summarized by the faculty member following the student presentations. Students are encouraged to discuss their perspectives on possible stressors and nursing interventions. This activity does not require a grade and has proven to be less stressful and more stimulating for students than a graded and longer presentation. This strategy actively involves the students in collaborative learning while providing an excellent review of the NSM. The primary purpose for the "mini presentation" is to give students practice in speaking and an opportunity for the faculty member to give positive feedback. Students view their peers as "experts" in at least one vital area of learning required of all of them, and the faculty member encourages students to consult their peers for information when caring for clients with similar diagnoses.

A second creative teaching strategy is implemented by faculty before the students' oral presentations. Faculty members model a previous student's care project. The student presents an individualized plan of care which meets needs of a client wholistically. The faculty member leads a discussion following the presentation, facilitating the process with open-ended questions about the case. A critique of the strong and weak points is summarized. It is common for students at this level in an associate degree program to concentrate on secondary interventions. Faculty suggest tertiary and primary interventions to expand thinking. Role-modeling occurs 2 weeks before student presentations so students can use the example to enhance their presentations.

A third teaching strategy encourages students to work with a mentor who can provide additional assistance and one-on-one guidance beyond that which is available during clinical time. Students frequently do an adequate job of gathering data using the assessment form. The Neuman Systems Model helps facilitate the organization of client data. However, diagnostic reasoning skills may be less developed. Mentors assist students to prioritize the problems based on the severity and penetration of the stressors. As students complete their nursing care projects, many are in Lewin's moving phase of implementing a change (Lewin, 1951).

Students are required to lead discussions following their oral presentations. Oral and written feedback from peers promotes collaborative learning. The student presenter has become a content expert on the specifics of the case, is able to answer most questions, and experiences increased self confidence speaking before peers. In subsequent weeks, students begin to utilize their peers for consultation.

Conclusions

Both faculty and students benefit from the implementation of strategies that promote critical thinking. As students develop the art of critical thinking, they are more likely to be able to perform with confidence and competence. Client responses are influential in identifying strategies effective in meeting their needs. Formative and summative evaluations between faculty and student provide direction and reinforce learning.

Nursing faculty benefit by collaboratively sharing effective teaching strategies in both class and clinical settings. A professional and collegial atmosphere promotes the growth of junior faculty members. Junior faculty are encouraged to ask questions and validate their ideas. Faculty have learned that they must be risk takers and try a variety of teaching strategies. Teachers sometimes believe there is minimal room for error in the teaching role; however, the IPFW faculty have discovered that it is much safer to try a new strategy in the classroom or during conference time than in the clinical setting when clients are involved. Our environment is conducive to learning by both students and faculty. The Neuman Systems Model provides the structure, and the strategies provide the process. Ultimately, the client benefits from comprehensive care provided by competent practitioners.

References

Anderson, L.W., & Sosniak, L.A. (Eds.). (1994). **Bloom's taxonomy: Forty year retrospective**. Chicago, IL: University of Chicago Press.

Jerit, L., & Taylor, B. (1992). Toward a definition of critical literacy. Des Plaines, IL: **Conference Proceedings of Critical Thinking/Critical Literacy**.

Lewin, K. (1951). **Field theory in social service**. New York: Harper

Neuman, B. (1995). **The Neuman Systems Model** (3rd ed.). Norwalk, CT: Appleton & Lange.

Chapter 5
Creative Teaching Strategies in a Neuman-Based Baccalaureate Curriculum
Priscilla Busch and Martha H. Lynch

Saint Anselm College is a Roman Catholic liberal arts college administered by the Benedictine monks of Saint Anselm Abbey and located in Southern New Hampshire. The college has earned national recognition for its unique approach to the study of the humanities. The core humanities curriculum seeks to give students a broad liberal arts education in a context of Christian ideals and serves as a solid foundation for later specialization.

The baccalaureate nursing program is committed to the "preparation of professional nurses who will function in ways which express Roman Catholic Christian values and ethics in the delivery of health care and the advancement of nursing science" (Nursing Department, 1986). In 1985, faculty members recognized the need for the curriculum to reflect current nursing education and practice. The Neuman Systems Model was selected as the conceptual framework for the curriculum because of its congruence with the philosophy and mission of the college and its wholistic view of the client as a composite of physiological, psychological, sociocultural, developmental, and spiritual variables (Neuman, 1989).

With the new curriculum ready for implementation, faculty members faced a dual challenge. First, they identified a need to develop teaching strategies designed to help students not only to learn the model but also to understand and use it in a meaningful way. Second, they selected strategies that stimulate problem-solving, to prepare students to function in today's changing health care system.

The National League for Nursing (1991) has also recognized this need and has charged nursing faculty with the task of preparing students to think critically. Nurses with baccalaureate degrees should be capable of using inductive and deductive reasoning to reach logical conclusions. Students need encouragement in use of alternative ways of thinking before arriving at conclusions. As Valiga (1988) states, "We need graduates who are able to be creative and willing to take risks" (p. 197). Educational approaches must be initiated both in classroom and clinical settings to achieve this outcome. Students need to experience diverse teaching strategies designed to enhance critical thinking and encourage creative problem solving. This chapter presents various approaches that have been initiated and used at Saint Anselm College to engage students in the teaching/learning process.

Curriculum Overview

The Nursing curriculum at Saint Anselm College begins in the sophomore year and builds on the core curriculum. Foundations of Nursing I and

II focus on primary prevention, health promotion, and development of the professional role. Junior year students examine stressors that threaten normal lines of defense. Emphasis in Dimensions of Nursing I & II is placed on primary and secondary prevention with some consideration for tertiary prevention. Content focuses on nursing care of the adult and the childbearing, child-rearing family. In Advanced Nursing I and II senior students address those nursing diagnoses that focus on collaborative problems and human responses to trauma, injury, violence, and psychosocial deficits. Students examine intrap-, inter-, and extra-personal variables that assist in attaining and maintaining client stability and integrity. Tertiary prevention is emphasized while primary and secondary preventions are reinforced. Nursing research, leadership, and management concepts are integrated throughout all nursing courses. Clinical practice is concurrent with theory and begins in Foundations of Nursing II. Students are placed in a variety of community, acute care, rehabilitation, and long-term care facilities.

The Neuman Systems Model provides a format for organizing class content and serves as a guide in clinical practice. If we expect students to use this framework in all phases of the nursing process, they must be familiar with every aspect of the model. To facilitate this process, faculty members need to use the Neuman vocabulary and consistently integrate the Neuman concepts and constructs into the theoretical content being addressed both in classroom and clinical settings. With consistent reinforcement, students "become Neumanized" and ready to use the model habitually.

Teaching The Model

Games. Gaming in its various forms is believed to be an effective method of obtaining and retaining information (Sprengel, 1994). Gaming approaches are pleasurable, remedial, and tension-reducing in nature. They offer opportunities to explore new and satisfying patterns of learning.

Implied in the concept of "Games" is a task to be accomplished and limits to be defined. Both structure and rules are clearly stated. Prizes for winners may or may not be given. Findings are shared with players when specific knowledge is acquired. Gaming allows students to be actively engaged in the learning process (Knowles, 1976). Individual behavioral and cognitive patterns may become apparent as the player processes the game. As the student becomes more self-aware, he/she may acknowledge and try out new behaviors and perhaps generalize them to other life situations. Games arise out of developmental needs and activities. The games we have chosen at Saint Anselm College reflect students' developmental and cognitive abilities and assist students in learning and applying the model.

Many students find the introduction of the Neuman Systems Model a challenge. Abstract concepts are difficult for some students to grasp. At Saint Anselm College, word puzzles are used to familiarize students with the vocabulary of the Neuman Systems Model. Word puzzles are familiar to most students and easy to learn. We found crossword puzzles to be an appropriate teaching/learning strategy for sophomore year students who are introduced to the Neuman Systems Model in the Fall Semester. Puzzles take on a straight-forward didactic approach to learning the model. They are meant not to be punitive or provocative, nor to be used as a testing device. Two forms of the puzzle have been developed (see **Figure 5.1 and 5.2**). With the help of the word list, most students are able to complete the puzzle with ease and experience a sense of achievement upon completion.

Figure 5.1: Puzzle A

Table 3
Puzzle A

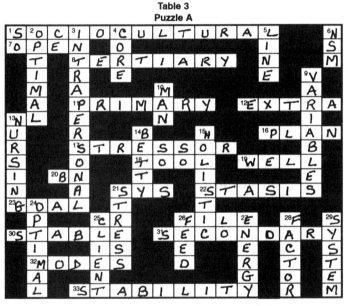

Word List

1. System
2. Nursing
3. Extra
4. Plan
5. Tertiary
6. Stress
7. Sociocultural
8. SYS
9. Core
10. Holistic
11. Optimal
12. Tool
13. Line
14. Goal
15. Intrapersonal
16. BN
17. Stressor
18. NSM
19. Well
20. Open
21. Optimal
22. Man
23. Client
24. Variables
25. Feed
26. Primary
27. File
28. Energy
29. Betty
30. CR
31. Modes
32. Factor
33. Stability
34. NL
35. STIC
36. Stasis
37. Secondary
38. Stable

Across

1. Variable - social & cultural functions
7. Continuous flow in input & process, output & feedback
8. Rehabilitation Group _____ Prevention
11. Prevention - Early case finding
12. Transfer from home to hospital, _____personal stressor
13. Normal Line (initials)
16. Patient Care _____
17. Disrupting environmental force
18. Facilities data gathering
19. Not ill
20. Founder of the Model (initials)
21. System (abbreviation)
22. Homeo_____
23. End product
25. Client Resources (initials)
26. To store data
30. Equilibrium
31. Treatment of symptoms prevention
32. Types or _____ of preventions
33. Balance and harmony

Down

2. State of Wellness - total person needs are met
3. Stressor - Interpersonal forces
4. Basic Structure
5. Normal _____ of defense
6. Neuman Systems Model (initials)
9. Physiological, Psychological, Sociocultural, Developmental, Spiritual
10. Person
13. Profession concerned with clients in their environment
14. Neuman (first name)
15. Wholistic (alternate spelling)
21. Tension producing stimuli
22. Systems Theory Illness Concept (Initials)
24. Best possible health state
25. Syn. with person
26. _____ back, provides for corrective action
27. Resources in the Basic Structure associated with Health/Illness
28. Intra, Inter, Extra personal stressor or _____
29. Client or client _____

Application of The Model

Throughout the curriculum, learning objectives reflect the use of the Neuman Systems Model. For example, in Dimensions of Nursing I, during a class on Modes of Prevention, a learning objective instructs students to examine potential stressors that may threaten a client with Diabetes Mellitus. A grid that lists the five Neuman variables in a vertical column and the intra-, inter-, and extra-personal variables horizontally is displayed on an overhead projector. This format stimulates problem-solving and discussion among students.

Figure 5.2: Puzzle B

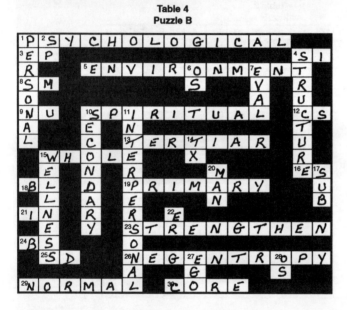

Table 4
Puzzle B

Word list

1. Primary
2. NU
3. Environment
4. Strengthen
5. Psychological
6. Wellness
7. Eval
8. Structure
9. SP
10. SUB
11. EP
12. Spiritual
13. Tertiary
14. Whole
15. SI
16. BS
17. Core
18. Negentropy
19. Man
20. CS
21. Normal
22. Interpersonal
23. EGO
24. ES
25. OS
26. Secondary
27. ER
28. SD
29. IN
30. Personal
31. TX
32. SM
33. BL

Across

1. Variable - mental processes & relationships
3. Stressor outside the person (initials)
4. Other initials for secondary prevention
5. Internal and external forces
8. Systems model (initials)
9. Nursing (abbreviation)
10. Variable associated with fostering hope
12. Client system (initials)
13. _____y prevention
15. The _____ not the parts
16. Tension producing forces in the environment (initials)
18. Boundary line (initials)
19. Intervention that strengthens flexible line of defense
21. Opposite of output (first syllable)
23. Goal _____ flexible line of defense
24. Basic Structure (initials)
25. Sensory deprivation (initials)
26. Energy conservation toward wellness
29. _____ line of Defense - standard for wellness deviance
30. Stability-_____ of the system

Down

1. Inter_____ factors
2. Reinstate stability level of intervention
4. Basic _____ or core
6. Organ strength (initials)
7. Last phase of the nursing process (abbreviation)
10. Intervention as treatment
11. Reinstate stability _____ prevention
14. Treatment (abbreviation)
15. _____ illness continuum
17. _____ part, not the whole
20. Person
22. Trauma site of secondary prevention (initials)
27. _____ structure - part of Basic Structure
28. Opposite of closed system (initials)

Similarly, in a class on Health Promotion, also given in Dimensions of Nursing I, objectives require students to identify variables that will influence response to hospitalization at each of a child's developmental stages and to formulate age-appropriate primary prevention strategies. Specific content deals with the stress of hospitalization on children. A list of the intra-, inter-, and extra-personal stressors which may threaten a young child's lines of defense are identified. A discussion of the multiple variables that protect lines of defense and activate lines of resistance follows.

Questioning Strategies. The use of questioning serves as an effective teaching tool to help students apply essential elements of the model to the content being presented (Wink, 1993). Using Bloom's Taxonomy as a theoretical framework, questions can be formulated to stimulate lower levels (knowledge or comprehension) or higher levels (application, analysis, synthesis, evaluation) of cognitive functioning (Wink, 1993). By questioning students, faculty members can determine if students are able to generalize previously acquired knowledge to new situations. This strategy also allows faculty to direct or redirect students' thinking process.

In the class on Modes of Prevention, the effects of diabetes on lifestyle of an individual are identified on the grid as extra-personal, developmental variables threatening the client. In this situation, an instructor asks a question to determine the depth of a student's knowledge (House, Chassie, & Spohn, 1990). Students are asked to compare how the lifestyle of a 42-year-old man, Type I diabetic, head of household, would differ from that of a 21-year-old, male, Type I, diabetic, college student. A well-formulated question enhances problem-solving and promotes participatory learning.

Similarly, in the class on Health Promotion—also presented in Dimensions of Nursing I—a faculty member asks students to identify primary prevention strategies appropriate for a hospitalized toddler and engages students in the learning activity. Once a comprehensive list of interventions has been examined, divergent questions are posed to stimulate analysis (House et al., 1990). Students are asked to discuss inherent variables that a 2 year old uses to activate lines of resistance and to compare these variables with those used by a 5 year old. Divergent questions stimulate higher order thinking because they encourage a variety of responses and require the learner to weigh information before drawing conclusions (House et al., 1990).

For example, in order to discuss variables that a toddler uses to respond to the stress of hospitalization, a student must first examine the intra-, inter-, and extra-personal variables related to separation anxiety and loss of control as stressors. Here, knowledge is required of the developmental variables influencing a toddler's versus a preschool child's behavioral responses. The lines of resistance expressed as negativism, regression, and temper tantrums may serve the toddler who is striving for autonomy. For the 5 year old, refusing to cooperate, physical aggressiveness, or fantasizing may also serve as a coping strategy.

Probing questions can also be used to extend the thinking process of students and to help them clarify or justify their conclusions (House et al., 1990; Wink, 1993). The length of time a faculty member waits after asking the question or after responding to a student's reply can influence the effectiveness of this technique. A wait time of 3 seconds or more gives the learner more processing time and facilitates increased student dialogue (Wink, 1993). We believe that questioning at appropriate times serves as an effective teaching strategy to facilitate student learning of the interventions in the Neuman Systems Model. Students must think when answering questions and are forced to apply knowledge to new situations.

Direct Analogy. Analogy is a form of reasoning in which similarities are inferred. This technique teaches students to connect their own personal experiences to what they are trying to learn. The art of thinking in analogies enhances synthesis and creative thinking because it encourages students to make connections through comparison. Direct analogy forces a student to compare the familiar with the unfamiliar and this process often leads to the discovery of something new through association. According to Gordon & Poze (1978) "learning by connection-making is efficient because it makes explicit the associative process by which the mind naturally assimilates knowledge" (p. 78).

Direct analogy has been used effectively in Dimensions of Nursing I and II to reinforce concepts from family systems theory by drawing on the analogy of the sport of bowling. Neuman views the family as having composite identity as well as an individual profile (Neuman, 1989). Students are instructed to compare family members to bowling pins. With guidance they begin to recognize the independence of the pins, as well as the interdependence of the set of pins to form a cohesive unit with system boundaries. Once a conceptual link between the pins and family members is made, students begin to view family dynamics in a new light. This metaphorical activity fosters reexamination of familiar concepts, expands students' thinking, and encourages them to explore new perspectives.

This analogy is then expanded by projecting the reactions of the pins as the bowling ball approaches. Some pins fall completely, some become unstable, yet manage to remain standing, while others appear untouched by the impact. Students are encouraged to speculate as to possible mechanisms responsible for shielding some pins while making others more vulnerable. This multidimensional response of the pins to the approaching ball is then likened to the reaction of family members (pins) to environmental stressors (ball) that can penetrate lines of defense. A brainstorming session follows, as students explore potential variables that play a role in strengthening or limiting the effectiveness of a family's lines of defense. This simple yet powerful analogy facilitates problem-solving and helps students develop a mental representation of family dynamics.

Personal Analogy. Personal analogy differs from direct analogy in that the participants are asked to compare themselves to an object or being.

Personal analogy challenges the affective domain by inviting students to use imagination in order to experience feelings. Students become emotionally engaged as they receive the following instructions.

Close your eyes, relax, and imagine for the next few minutes that you are an anniversary clock. You sit majestically on an exquisite cherry mantle where you have resided for many years. A sparkling glass dome, which is kept meticulously clean, covers your body. Your shining equidistant spheres never fail to oscillate, as your two hands move synchronously and rhythmically. You are often the center of attention in this room; people consult you frequently throughout the day. Suddenly, without warning, an intruder begins to lift your dome and it drops to the floor and shatters.

Again, students are instructed to assume the identity of the clock. They are given a few minutes to experience this role, then asked to describe "How do I feel now as I sit on the mantle?" As students share this experience, responses are listed on the blackboard. Frequently reports include, "vulnerable, anxious, nervous, angry, cold, scared." When a variety of responses have been expressed, faculty members begin to relate the feelings and emotions expressed by students to the feelings clients often experience when their lines of defense have been penetrated.

We believe direct and personal analogies to be effective teaching strategies for all learners. Analogies force students to consider situations from an alternative perspective. This technique enhances problem-solving and creative expression on the part of students.

Simulation Games. Simulation is a role-playing situation that relates to real life experiences. The purpose of using simulation is to reinforce present knowledge as well as previously learned information (Hanna, 1994). Simulation helps students use the Neuman Systems Model to address clinical problems and serves as an effective teaching strategy for students who are entering clinical practice. In simulation, a case study is provided as the teaching tool. This game is appropriate for small group interaction. Players are randomly divided into either two or three competing teams made up of two to six students each. Each competing team has an assigned recorder. Yet another team, called the audience challenge team, is made up of the remainder of the students. All students are involved with specific tasks at a variety of performance levels.

A time keeper is assigned from the audience challenge team. All team members are given a case study to read as shown in **Table 5.1**. (Other case studies of varying complexity can be used to address different student levels.) Recorders from the competing teams record either on a chalk board or on a form that lists the five Neuman variables and the three stressor sources derived from the case study. Examples from the five variables and three stressors could include: physical injuries, somatic complaints, sleep deprivation, and heavy alcohol use as evidence of physiological variables. Psychological variables are illustrated with Mrs. Barton's expressed sadness, denial of the situation by Mr. Barton, and somatic complaints plus hyper-

Table 5.1: Case Study

Jan Barton is a slightly obese, disheveled-appearing 31-year-old married woman, the mother of three children: Ann, age 6; Torry, age 18 months; and Jennifer, age 6 months. She was brought to the emergency department by her 42-year-old husband, Jason, an unemployed truck driver. The family has recently relocated in the hope that Mr. Barton will find employment.

Mrs. Barton has a 3-cm cut on her left mandible and two fresh bruises on her lower abdomen. The smell of alcohol lingers about the couple.

Mr. Barton is quick to speak for his wife explaining that her injuries were the result of slipping on a scatter rug in the kitchen. He hopes that her injuries will be attended promptly because the children were left behind in the care of a neighbor, a 70-year-old woman who is visually impaired. "We need to get home so that we can get back to normal," he added.

While Mrs. Barton's cut is being sutured she begins to cry. "Don't mind me," she tells the nurse, "I cry all the time I'm so tired, I never get much sleep." She explains that baby Jennifer still wakes up several times a night for a bottle. She describes Torry as "a demon on wheels," on the go all day long. Ann, the 6 year old, has lately been refusing to attend school complaining of stomach aches. Mrs. Barton admits tolerating her husband's heavy alcohol use because she's afraid that he will walk out on the family. She denies that he physically abuses her or that alcohol is a problem for her. Mrs. Barton admits feeling overwhelmed.

activity in the children. Sociocultural variables would include: the family relocating to a new city, financial problems, and lack of support. Developmental variables are demonstrated inherently in the children's individual developmental needs and Mr. Barton's unemployment status. Spiritual variables are reflected in Mrs. Barton's feeling of being overwhelmed, having "no where to turn," fear of abandonment, and discouragement about heavy alcohol use by the husband. Instances of intra-personal stressors could include losses, emotional pain, exhaustion, fear of abandonment. Inter-personal stressors are demonstrated in the question of physical abuse, alcohol abuse, poor communication, fear, and limited support. Extra-personal stressors are reflected in Mr. Barton's status of being unemployed and the stress of relocation.

At the end of 5 minutes, time is called by the time keeper. The audience challenge team then has opportunity for rebuttal and may challenge the selection and placement of stressors. The team with the most correct answers is declared the winner. Faculty input and final consensus from the players determine the winning team. No prizes are awarded. We believe this keeps competition at a suitable level (Bloom & Trice, 1994).

We have used simulation games to supplement classroom content and to prepare students for clinical experience. Simulation games actively involve participants in the learning process and provide a practical experience in preparation for real clinical situations.

Clinical Journaling. Clinical journaling is yet another way of reinforcing use of the Neuman Systems Model in the clinical setting and helping students develop critical thinking skills. At one level, journaling is simply a written record of events. However, as a student interacts with the journal, by recording, reading, and sharing its content with a clinical faculty member, the journal can become a powerful learning tool (Hahnemann, 1986).

Journaling can become a means for deepening of insights, experiencing process, improving conceptualization, and discovering personal dimensions. Because reactions to events vary greatly from person to person and context to context, the interpretation of events often determines how students will proceed. Learning may occur quite differently depending upon one's reaction and interpretation of events.

Journaling places considerable responsibility on students, yet students are not alone in getting their learning and affective needs met. A dialogue with internal and external components occurs in the journaling process. Personal feedback occurs from the student's internal dialogue and from external sources. The clinical faculty member's comments to the student make up the external source. After incorporating internal and external feedback, the student is encouraged to practice new behaviors if indicated and to obtain feedback from faculty on the degree to which his or her behavior produces the intended outcome.

For example, a young male client in his early teens made a derogatory remark regarding a student nurse's weight. The student wrote in her journal of the humiliation, anger, and desire to counter the emotional injury and registered her hope that the client would be discharged before another encounter occurred. External feedback was promptly provided by the clinical faculty member. The student was commended for her emotional honesty. She was supported empathetically and provided with alternative approaches to try with clients who speak inappropriately. A discussion of the client's intra-, inter-, and extra-personal stressors provided a wholistic understanding of the behavior exhibited.

Journaling provides for a wide range of learning opportunities. Learning occurs through mutual sharing of situations not readily observable by others, so a wider range of a learner's resources are developed. Students can increase competencies of knowing, valuing, and choosing future actions.

A simplified version of journaling is appropriate for students entering the clinical area for the first time. By carefully structuring the clinical assignment, students begin to apply theory to clinical practice. For example, the objective for a given clinical assignment might be "identifying physiological, psychological, and developmental variables that will alter the nutritional progress of the child or adult." This assignment clearly directs students to the specific data to be collected and examined. Journaling then provides the forum for discussion of assessment and evaluation. Through faculty and student dialogue students receive individual feedback and learn to examine critically their perceptions and observations (Burnard, 1988).

A clinical journal chart is used by senior-year students. These students are asked to keep a journal of their clinical experiences. Students are instructed to review and record on the form provided (see **Table 5.2**) interac-

Table 5.2: Clinical Journaling

Keeping a journal is a way of organizing and examining one's clinical experiences so as to enhance learning. Please review and record your interactions with clients, staff, faculty, and peers. Keep in mind Physiological, Psychological, Sociocultural, Spiritual, and Developmental variables and the intra-, inter-, and extra-personal stressors as utilized in the Neuman Systems Model. When completed, please return to the appropriate clinical faculty member. Feedback will be provided.

What Happened? Why?
Describe the event: The individual(s) involved;
their verbal/nonverbal behavior.

My reaction;
What I felt;
Physical cues;
Who or what was involved?

What I have learned:
Striking thoughts, insights;
new behavior(s).

tions with clients, staff, faculty, and peers and to address Neuman's schema of five variables and three stressors. Students return the completed form to their clinical faculty member. The faculty member reads, writes comments, and returns the form to the students. Students are asked to retain the form until the end of the clinical rotation, when students are encouraged to use the completed journal in writing their self-evaluations.

Conclusion

We have presented a repertoire of teaching and learning techniques that we believe enhance critical thinking by actively engaging students in the teaching-learning process. Although these strategies have been successfully integrated into our curriculum, they are consistently being refined for application at each student level. Alternative approaches to journaling are also being tested as faculty members make the transition from the traditional inpatient supervision role to community-based learning. As our teaching methods become more sophisticated we can begin to initiate strategies to integrate the Neuman Systems Model into our research and community service role.

We hope that these creative approaches will stimulate other educators to consider ways that will facilitate internalization of the Neuman Systems Model as well as enhance critical thinking in students.

References

Bloom, K., & Trice, L. (1994). Let the games begin. **The Journal of Nursing Education, 33**(4), 151-152.

Burnard, P. (1988). The journal as an assessment and evaluation tool in nursing education. **Nurse Education Today, 8**, 105-107.

Gordon, W., & Poze, T. (1978). Learning dysfunction and connection making. **Psychiatric Annals, 8**(3), 140-145.

Hahnemann, B. (1986). Journal writing: A key to promoting critical thinking in nursing students. **Journal of Nursing Education, 25**(5), 213-215.

Hanna, D. (1994). Using simulation to teach clinical nursing. **Nurse Educator, 16**(2), 28-30.

House, B., Chassie, M., & Spohn, B. (1990). Questioning: An essential ingredient in effective teaching. **The Journal of Continuing Education in Nursing, 21**(5), 196-201.

Knowles, M.S. (1976). **The modern practice of adult education: Andragogy versus pedagogy.** New York: Associated Press.

National League for Nursing. (1991). **Criteria for the evaluation of baccalaureate and higher degree programs in nursing** (6th ed.). New York: NLN.

Neuman, B. (1989). **The Neuman Systems Model (2nd ed.).** Norwalk, CT: Appleton & Lange.

Nursing Department, Manchester, NH: Saint Anselm College. (1986). Nursing Department Philosophy.

Sprengel, A. (1994). Learning can be fun with gaming. **The Journal of Nursing Education, 33**(4), 151-152.

Wink, D. (1993). Using questioning as a teaching strategy. **Nurse Educator, 18**(5), 11-15.

Valiga, T.M. (1988). Curriculum outcomes and cognitive development: New perspectives for nursing education. In E. Bevis & J. Watson (Eds.), **Curriculum Revolution: Mandate for change.** New York: National League for Nursing.

Chapter 6
Critical Thinking Strategies for Family and Community Client Systems
Janet S. Hassell

Lander University School of Nursing, located in semi-rural Greenwood, South Carolina, offers a 4-year, liberal arts nursing education program based on the Neuman Systems Model (NSM). The NSM was adopted by nursing faculty in 1988 at the time of transition from a 2-year associate degree nursing program to the present 4-year baccalaureate degree program. Reasons cited by faculty for the selection of the NSM included its wholistic, systems-based framework and its compatibility with the human needs and stress adaptation concepts used at the associate degree level (Sipple & Freese, 1989).

In the Lander University nursing curriculum, students are introduced to the general concept of nursing models and the NSM at the sophomore level (Level I). In Level II, students focus on individuals as clients in the context of families, groups, or communities. In Level III, the focus broadens to include the mother-child dyad, the family-as-client, and the community-as-client. These concepts are included in the community/public health nursing course, a required component of the baccalaureate nursing curriculum, before a semester of synthesis of the nursing program (Level IV). Throughout the curriculum, the NSM serves as an effective organizational structure that facilitates the development of critical thinking skills.

Critical thinkers examine assumptions, concepts, empirical information, inferences, implications and consequences, alternative viewpoints, and frames of reference as processes of reasoned, problem-solving thought. The NSM is an effective organizational structure that facilitates the development of critical thinking skills. As the model is used for assessing client systems, students learn to think with universal principles that transcend client differences.

The complexity of community-as-client concepts provides multiple opportunities for both model application and critical thinking. Through discussion and modeling by instructors, students gain skill in applying Neuman concepts to actual situations. During class time, student groups analyze community and aggregate assessment data to practice identifying stressors, degrees of response, and lines of defense for complex client systems such as residents of a high-rise apartment building for elders, the homeless in a downtown ghetto, or adolescents in a high school.

Through the use of Neuman-based assessment tools, students collect data, then plan and evaluate interventions in their clinical field experiences. Early in the semester, students select a pregnant or recent postpartum client for home visits. Initially, students use model concepts to develop individual-focused care within the context of the childbearing family. Students use an individual assessment tool adapted by their instructor from Neuman (1989) and Bates (1991) to structure their approach to individual clients for accurate information collection. The basic core of the selected client is assessed, as well as other interactive systems such as the dynamics of the mother-child dyad. From these assessments, normal lines of defense, flexible lines of defense, and lines of resistance are derived. Stressors to the mother, such as hormonal and body image changes, sibling rivalry, and limits on sexual activity are identified. The degree of reaction to stressors is assessed, and problems—stated as nursing diagnoses—defined. Interventions are designed to resolve problems for the individual client within the context of the family and community.

Whole Families

Students then broaden their focus from the identified individual or mother-child dyad in the child-bearing family to the whole family-as-client system. A Neuman-based family assessment tool adapted by their instructor from Reed (1989) and Friedman (1992) helps students organize data as physiological, psychological, sociocultural, developmental, and spiritual variables from the family-as-client perspective. Assessment of the family-as-client requires students to focus on group dynamics, communication, power relationships, stress and crisis management, social and cultural influences, and the general health of the family. In these applications, students must define and analyze the effects of stressors on variables from a family perspective. Stressors such as isolation, increased economic hardship, abuse, physical violence, and lack of access to services are identified by analyzing interactions of individuals within family boundaries, with consideration of developmental stages of the family influenced by sociocultural factors. Interventions are designed to relieve identified family stressors and to emphasize family strengths, encouraging use of their unique characteristics to regain cohesiveness, develop coping skills, and reduce isolation. As students suggest community resources, families increase their access to health care systems, to education and/or economic resources such as Aid to Families with Dependent Children (AFDC), or to job training. Through comprehensive assessments, stressor and strength identification, and proposed intervention strategies, students use higher level, critical thinking skills.

Using the basic core as an example, **Table 6.1** illustrates the change of assessment focus required as the client system increases in complexity from the individual to the community. The strength and flexibility of the model is demonstrated as students identify aspects of the five variables within several client systems.

This grid demonstrates how students can cluster data and interpret cues, leading to synthesis of information in nursing diagnoses and plans of care. Each of these mental processes is a critical thinking skill. Faculty guide and refine cognitive processes through role modeling and feedback that reinforces and validates the student's critical thinking skills. The examples that

Table 6.1: Assessing Basic Core Components in Various Clients

Component	Individual	Family	Community
Physiological:	Vital signs, height, weight, medical hx., immune status, lab values, nutrition, general health. Health habits. Health care, risk factors.	Hereditary disease, risk factors, impact of living environment on physical health, family diet & nutritional status, patterns of activity and rest, general health.	Vital statistics, other morbidity/mortality data, risk factors, immunity status, environmental influences on physical & emotional health, safety, violence, drugs, available services.
Sociocultural:	Ethnic/cultural issues, language, socioeconomic status, customs/taboos of food/health/illness, time orientation, sex roles, education level, access to health care, personal mobility, degree of isolation.	Ethnic/cultural influences on family roles, group dynamics, power/control relationships, language barriers, child-rearing practices, access to services and health care, communication.	Demographic profile, education level, dominant subcultures, economic status, mobility, isolation, general lifestyle, cultural values, attitudes toward vulnerable populations, political structures, funding sources.
Psychological:	Attitudes, values, self-image, self esteem, coping skills, cognitive abilities, emotional health, anxiety level.	Intermember affective support, coping skills, communication patterns, common health beliefs.	Emotional health, values, prevalence of divorce, fear, violence, world view, political mood, self vs. society orientation.
Developmental:	Developmental stage Status of developmental tasks completion, problems.	Developmental stage Significant life events Maturational crises.	Evolutionary stage of community (new, developing, established, decaying).
Spiritual:	Religious beliefs, tenets Spiritual values. Congruence of values with family & community.	Spiritual influence within family unit.culture. Congruence with the community.	Predominant religious culture. Spiritual values. Congruence with sub-cultures, other communities.
Intersystem Variables:	Intra-personal: within the individual Inter-personal: between persons, same as intrafamily boundaries.	Intrafamily: Interaction among members. Interfamily: Interaction with societal systems, influenced by family boundaries.	Intracommunity: Health/safety systems Cultural systems. Educational systems. Communication systems. Transportation systems. Economic systems. Recreation, Law, Politics, Spiritual, & Religious systems.

Adapted from Anderson et al., (1986), Beddome (1989), Reed (1989), and Friedman (1992).

follow illustrate how students develop critical thinking skills through the application of the NSM to individual, family, and community client systems in a Level III community health nursing course at Lander University.

In the first example, a student accompanied a community health nurse on a home visit to a school-age boy with an open, infected wound on his foot. After assessing the child and the family context within which he lived, the student identified appropriate nursing diagnoses, (a) impaired skin integrity related to effects of injury to right foot, as evidenced by open wound and drainage; (b) knowledge deficit related to not recognizing signs and symptoms of infection, as evidenced by father's and patient's self-reports; and (c) potential infection related to poor water quality in home (Barnes, 1994). Interventions included traditional task-related elements of wound care but also reflected the family and community context, identifying specific roles of the client and family members in the care of the wound, and health promotion and prevention by teaching self-care skills. Referrals of the family were made for financial assistance and analysis of the water supply. This example illustrates development of critical thinking skills in serving an individual in a home setting.

In a second example, a 40-year-old nursing student assessed her own family and described a normal line of defense characterized by no acute or chronic disease, inadequate health practices such as smoking, high fat diet, and lack of exercise, middle age, a positive outlook on life countered by considerable stress related to wife's college commitments, mutual dependence yet frequent career conflicts, and a strong faith in a higher being (Phillips, 1994). Lines of resistance were described as a three-generation support system and mature perceptions through experience of what constitutes a stressor. Flexible lines of defense were described as resilient, based on maturity, strong interpersonal relationships, and accurate anticipation of the effects of stressors on their lives. The family nursing diagnoses and problem statements identified by the student included:

1. Altered health maintenance related to inadequate health practices as evidenced by smoking, high fat diet, and lack of exercise.

2. Lack of intimacy related to dissimilar schedules and fatigue as evidenced by having meals together only on weekends, going to bed at different times, and not being able to experience social activities together.

3. High risk for impaired normal line of defense related to positive family history of heart attacks and lung cancer.

4. Decisional conflicts related to careers as evidenced by anxiety and worry over outcomes of decisions.

5. Altered spiritual interaction related to work as evidenced by irregular church attendance.

6. Potential for anxiety related to financial crises, health changes in elderly parents, and effects of aging.

7. Potential for ineffective coping related to physical signs of aging, aging parents, and disruption of emotional bonds secondary to lack of time.

In the above example, the student used critical thinking to analyze the data, thus listing family strengths and areas for improvement as evidenced by the diagnoses. Family-focused interventions of sensible lifestyle changes and stress management strategies were built on the assessed strengths of the family's normal line of defense, lines of resistance, flexible lines of defense, and stressors.

Community Assessment

The Community Assessment Group Project is a major activity of this community health nursing course and reflects the importance of community assessments to community/public health nursing practice. The community assessment project represents the next higher level of client complexity and assists students to understand the concept of population-based or aggregate-based nursing.

Students use a community assessment tool based on the Community-As-Client Model adapted from the Neuman Systems Model by Anderson, McFarlane, and Helton (1986) to organize data into basic core, interdependent subsystems, and external environment systems. This NSM-based community assessment prompts students to use higher level, abstract thought to consider the dynamic interactions among individuals, families, groups, variables, and contexts that define communities.

Students work in small groups and assess aggregate, geopolitical, or other communities. They are encouraged by the faculty to select aggregates or communities in which they have interest, experience, or concern. When faculty are aware of unique situations or circumstances in the general community that warrant assessment, students are encouraged to select this aggregate or community as a project. An example of such a situation was a diphtheria epidemic in a three-county area, involving an aggregate of approximately 150 infected persons. Students worked with local public health nurses and were assisted by faculty to assess this unique aggregate.

Other examples of communities and aggregates selected by students have included smokers and non-smokers on a university campus, an aggregate population of women in a college dormitory, the aggregate population of tuberculosis cases within a health district, an aggregate population of persons at risk for rabies in South Carolina, pregnant women at risk for AIDS in a community, the migrant population in a South Carolina county, highway patrol officers in a South Carolina district, homeless people in a southern city, and elderly people at a nursing home.

In addition to assessing the basic core of these groups, intersystem variables and external environmental variables are also assessed for stressors. Critical thinking is necessary to analyze, synthesize, and derive community problem statements or nursing diagnoses from the data as supported by evidence. For example, the students who examined the South Carolina population at risk for rabies determined that South Carolina has a strong normal line of defense, with lines of resistance represented by legal guidelines for public health and veterinarian duties, epidemiologic studies of rabies in South Carolina, and wildlife control programs. Flexible lines of defense were represented by low-cost rabies clinics and occasional education programs. However, increases in confirmed rabies cases concurrent with other identified factors prompted the students to make a community nursing diagnosis of "infection transmission, high risk for rabies related to non-compliance with pet immunization programs, and exposure to infected wildlife" (Dixon, Mollison, Myers, Sims, Gardner, & Koller, 1994).

In addition, students determined that "a combination of stressors: increased rate of rabies, large rural population, high illiteracy rate, high incidence of animal bites in children, and limited funding lead to a population at risk for rabies and in need of an accurate, easy-to-understand and cost-efficient rabies education program" (Dixon et al., 1994). A second community nursing diagnosis generated from this assessment was "knowledge deficit related to transmission of rabies, symptoms of rabies, animal avoidance tactics, immunization, and rabies treatment, as evidenced by increased animal quarantine rates, increased non-pet-bite investigations, and pet-bite investigations" (Dixon et al., 1994).

In the above example, students developed innovative interventions aimed at children in the population. Dog and cat character puppets, billboards, and school-based education programs carried a message to encourage improved rates of cat and dog immunization against rabies. As required of all students in this course, projects were shared with classmates during in-class presentations.

As seen from the preceding examples, students in a community health nursing course are able to use the Neuman Systems Model at various levels of client-system complexity to organize data, analyze, reason, draw conclusions, and propose problem solutions through critical thinking. The assessment of individuals in family and community health contexts prompts students to consider the implications and consequences of interventions in relation to the economic, social, and health status of the larger community in which the families live. Students learn that access to community health services is significantly determined by political and ideological systems interacting with client systems.

As a result, students learn to broaden the focus of their nursing interventions to consider enabling interactions with individual clients and client families that incorporate multidisciplinary involvement and case management activities. This broader focus facilitates students' critical thinking skills by identifying and initiating problem solving strategies that extend beyond traditional nursing boundaries to address community-based problems at their source.

References

Anderson, E., McFarlane, J., & Helton, A. (1986). Community-as-client: A model for practice. **Nursing Outlook, 5(34)**, 220-223.

Barnes, T. (1994). **Nursing care plan**. Unpublished manuscript.

Bates, B. (1991). **A guide to physical examination and history taking** (5th ed.). Philadelphia, PA: Lippincott.

Beddome, G. (1989). Application of the Neuman Systems Model to the assessment of community-as-client. In B. Neuman (Ed.), **The Neuman Systems Model** (2nd ed.). Norwalk, CT: Appleton & Lange.

Dixon, T., Mollison, K., Myers, L., Sims, V., Gardner, M., & Koller, L. (1994). **Rabies in South Carolina: A community assessment**. Unpublished manuscript.

Neuman, B. (1989). **The Neuman Systems Model** (2nd ed.). Norwalk, CT: Appleton & Lange.

Friedman, M. (1992). **Family nursing: Theory and practice**. Norwalk, CT: Appleton & Lange.

Phillips, N. (1994). **Nursing care plan**. Unpublished manuscript.

Reed, K. (1989). Family theory related to the Neuman Systems Model. In B. Neuman (Ed.), **The Neuman Systems Model** (2nd ed.). Norwalk, CT: Appleton & Lange.

Sipple, J.A., & Freese, B.T. (1989). Transition from technical to professional-level nursing education. In B. Neuman (Ed.), **The Neuman Systems Model** (2nd ed.). Norwalk, CT: Appleton & Lange.

Chapter 7
The Neuman Systems Model, Critical Thinking, and Cooperative Learning in a Nursing Issues Course
Opal A. Freiburger

After several semesters of teaching an "issues in nursing" course to second-level students in an associate degree nursing program at Indiana University-Purdue University at Fort Wayne, I began to experiment with strategies designed to encourage student participation and stimulate interest in the course. Some students were quite vocal about their opinions that this two-credit required course would be of little value to them in nursing. Their major interests were task-oriented nursing skills and learning new techniques rather than broader aspects of healthcare issues. Feedback from students simulated that of "received knowers" (Belenky, Clinchy, Goldberger, & Tarule, 1986, pp. 36-43). Students wanted "more structure" to be given the required information without understanding or evaluating an idea. They also asked the teacher to, "Tell me what you want me to know." "Tell me what I need to know to pass the exams." In response to the use of small-group methods, students initially voiced concern that the small-group activity would not prepare them for determining the "right" answers for test questions. Students thought lectures were a better method for teaching this content.

A major teaching goal became development of a course of action designed to encourage students to actively participate in small groups and be receptive to sharing their knowledge, experiences, and thoughts with other students in order to maximize their own learning and that of others. This outcome was reflected in the comment of a college junior, "This year I realized that I can use my mind," (Belenky et al., 1986, p. 87) and the teacher may ask, "How can the educator facilitate the ability of students to recognize and cultivate their intellectual processes [before] their junior year in college?"

Bruffee (1995) refers to teachers as cultural agents who promote reacculturation to learning through associations with others. He advocates learning to share "our toys" (our books, ideas, beliefs, way of life, country, and world) and states that doing so is a lifelong venture (p. 13). Changing students' attitudes so they place higher value on education and embrace self-disciplined learning is facilitated by small-group activities in which students interact, influencing each other's perceptions (Johnson, Johnson, & Smith, 1991, p. 6:13). Utilizing qualities of critical thinking was identified as a format for providing guidelines and encouraging students to engage in processes of group learning. Thus, the Neuman Systems Model became the basis for integrating critical thinking and cooperative learning into the nursing issues course.

Neuman Systems Model Application

The Neuman Systems Model is the theoretical framework for the design of the course. Basic concepts of the model are included in the course manual as reference material. Course content is categorized as primarily intra-, inter-, or extra-personal relevant to nurses, nurses' role, the nursing profession, the larger society, or the nursing issue being discussed for that class period.

The purpose of the nursing issues course is to assist students make an effective transition from the role of student to that of a registered nurse. Classes for the two-credit course meet weekly for 2 hours. The course is designed to encourage students to think critically, be an active participant, share experiences, learn from each other, explore the thinking of all participants, incorporate concepts of the Neuman Systems Model, and respect the rights of others.

To facilitate application of the model, "Inquiries for Application of the Neuman Systems Model," was developed. This tool assists students to address major aspects of the model when considering a nursing issue. These inquiries reflect major stressors of the issue, the usual state of equilibrium for the situation, factors that may weaken the normal line of defense, actions to prevent penetration of the normal line of defense, and available factors that may aid in protecting the core (Neuman, 1995, pp. 16-37). Each area of content is introduced by a diagram that reflects a relationship among stressors, stabilizing forces (flexible and normal lines of defense and lines of resistance), the content, and the perspective from which the content will be addressed (intra-, inter-, or extra-personal).

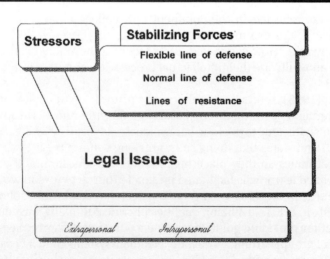

Figure 7.1: Relationship among stressors, stabilizing forces, and content

Course content includes such topics as the history of nursing, critical thinking, the image of nursing, nursing education, healthcare delivery, political action in nursing, ethical issues, conflict management, nursing licensure, legal issues, wholistic health strategies for nurses, and employment.

Discussion questions and specific assignments are given for each of the content areas that are addressed during the semester. Questions must reflect application of the Neuman Systems Model. Students are encouraged to add questions for class discussion and space is available in the manual for that purpose. The course manual also includes general information about the course, teaching methodology, grading system, and handout materials.

Sample questions in Freiburger's 1995-1996 course manual to assist students in preparing for class discussions include: (a) What survival factors have been integrated into the basic structure (core) of nursing through the course of history? (b) How does the profession interact with its internal and external environment? (c) What stressors have been imposed on the profession relevant to the various types of nursing programs for entry into practice? (d) What techniques can the nurse use to promote stability of the system through assertive communication? (e) What practices may be implemented to protect nurses from stress of a legal nature? (f) What stressors are you experiencing that are within the buffer zone of your flexible line of defense?

Creating a Cooperative Learning Environment

Creating a system for learning which promotes a free exchange of knowledge, perceptions, and speculations within a group is a challenge for both the students and faculty. Students must be willing to share their ideas and assume risks of self-disclosure to actively participate in the group process. Through active involvement students reveal their ability to articulate thoughts, explore new ideas, and examine their perceptions in light of group constructed knowledge. They must respect the rights of others to express, discuss, and compare views which may be different from their own. Students are exposed to intra-, inter-, and extra-personal stressors which may result from concerns about self-disclosure, conflicts, and the pressure of meeting course requirements. In response to group interactions, such stressors may affect the flexible line of defense to the extent that normal lines of defense of group processes are threatened. Thus, participants must collectively maintain established standards for effective group functioning to preserve the integrity of the system. The faculty member, the key player in establishing the climate for learning, must be willing to recognize the active role of students in constructing knowledge. The educator is responsible for promoting educational opportunities that focus on the cultivation of competencies and talents of students.

An unexpected event that occurred when the author implemented a new teaching strategy exemplifies situations that may be encountered when new techniques are introduced in the classroom. Students had been verbally assigned to write about the following for class: (a) describe a stressful situation experienced in nursing; (b) on a second piece of paper, describe your response to the situation, and (c) identify strategies that could have been used to decrease your stress in the situation. The plan, which the teacher thought was clearly presented the previous week, was to give each student's paper describing the stressful situation anonymously to a peer. The peer was asked to write suggestions for responding to the stressful situation. Discussion of the stressful situation and a peer's suggested response to it was to follow with the anonymity of the student who had experienced the situation maintained. The student's actual response and retrospective assessment of strategies to reduce stress in the situation would not be shared with other students.

During class, however, several students objected to discussing the stressful experiences. Consequently, the faculty proposed that sharing the stressful situation for discussion would be voluntary. The papers with the stressful situation and comments from a peer were then returned to the student who had originally submitted the stressful situation. The response to the teacher's proposal was favorable and students voluntarily presented stressful experiences for class discussion. A very helpful discussion of actual stressful situations ensued.

This unique and valued learning experience reflects the need for faculty to give clear instructions, be flexible, be sensitive, respect students, nurture student-faculty relationships, and model professional behaviors which promote group processes. Interestingly, the experience tended to augment group process activities for the remainder of the semester and the teaching strategy has been successfully incorporated into the nursing issues course.

Critical-thinking concepts are introduced to students in the nursing issues course through the use of a videotape, "Thinking Towards Decisions" (Chaffee, 1989). The videotape exemplifies the use of small-group participation in discussing elements of critical thinking that are depicted in a simulated situation. Students in the issues class have an opportunity to participate in discussions at intervals during the presentation and to compare their responses with those of the students featured on the videotape.

Qualities of critical thinking that are emphasized in the nursing issues course include: thinking actively, carefully exploring issues, supporting viewpoints with reasons, thinking autonomously, taking different perspectives, engaging in dialogue, being receptive, and using reasoned judgment (Chaffee, 1990, pp. 37-93). Students are encouraged to apply these qualities of critical thinking in all aspects of the class: small group discussions, self-assessments, examinations, and other written assignments. These qualities of critical thinking formulate the criteria for grading papers. Students are asked not only to apply but also to identify what qualities of critical thinking were used in the described situation. A sample examination question may be, "Describe an experience you have had in nursing and discuss how critical thinking was, or could have been, applied in that situation. Identify the quality of critical thinking you use and support your viewpoints."

Students are required to complete two self-assessments during a semester. On both assessments students rate their abilities to use critical thinking and their performance in group functioning roles. The first self-assessment tool includes goal statements for improving class participation and critical thinking skills and citation of an example of how the Neuman Systems Model was applied in clinical practice. For the second self-assessment the student evaluates the attainment of goals from the first assessment and is expected to give specific examples for the use of self-evaluation for professional development in clinical nursing practice.

Student and Faculty Responses to Changes in the Issues Course

Extensive experimentation with teaching strategies and content areas over a 4-year period culminated in the development of the first manual for an Issues in Nursing course. The innovative use of the Neuman Systems Model as the integrating theoretical framework for the application of critical thinking and cooperative learning to the nursing issues course has been an effective and rewarding endeavor. Overall, student responses have been increasingly favorable to the multiple teaching tools and techniques that have been implemented. Students tend to view the manual as providing a more comprehensive and structured approach for the issues course. They have the opportunity to offer input in decision-making about such items as the dates for exams and deadlines for papers.

Students have given meaningful feedback which has been instrumental in shaping many aspects of the course. For example, when the course was first taught, the examinations were largely content-oriented multiple choice questions. Yet, the overwhelming question was, "How are students applying the course content to their individual experiences in clinical practice?" Self-response (short answer) items were incorporated into examinations in an effort to learn more about the students' thinking processes and their application of theory to practice. With the addition of a number of self-response items, students complained that the exams were "too long." They made a valid point. Unexpectedly, many students tended to give extensive responses to these items.

Several revisions that were made simultaneously resolved the problem and produced positive results. These course revisions included: a take-home component for each exam, a reduction of the number of self-response items on the in-class exams, and specific criteria for each self-response item. Students have voiced an increased desire for use of the self-response items and the take-home exams. An example of a take-home exam item might be to (a) "Identify at least one stressor that you have experienced or expect to experience as a new registered nurse in the clinical setting" and (b) "Discuss what strategies could be used to reduce the stressor(s)."

Students' responses to questions about relating course content to experiences they have had or witnessed in the clinical setting have been very enlightening. For instance, the exam item might request identifying a clinical experience and discuss how critical or creative thinking was, or could have been, applied. Students often respond by describing an experience they have had and addressing how it could have been improved. This type of activity tends to facilitate self evaluation and promote strategies that enhance professional development. Perhaps students' receptivity to self-response types of exam items is nurtured by their need and desire to "tell their stories." Evidence points in that direction.

Using the Neuman Systems Model to create a nursing issues course integrating critical thinking and cooperative learning continues to be a challenging and rewarding endeavor. As experimentation continues and new teaching-learning strategies for the course are tested and refined, one must heed the claim that, "Gaining expertise in using cooperative learning takes at least one lifetime" (Johnson et al., 1991, p. 10:10). Yet, one must also savor such students' evaluation comments as: "This class wasn't as boring as I thought it would be." and "The issues we've discussed in class have broadened my horizons and opened my eyes."

Ultimately, faculty-student interactions create and shape shared, reciprocal, educational experiences for faculty and students. We learn from, and with, each other. Such student-faculty interaction is the hallmark of the educative-caring paradigm. It is critical to begin this educational process at the first level of nursing education if we are to produce technically competent nurses who are educated rather than trained.

References

Belenky, M.F., Clinchy, B.M., Goldberger, R.R., & Tarule, J.M. (1986). **Women's ways of knowing: the development of self, voice, and mind**. New York: Basic Books.

Bruffee, K.A. (1995, January/February). Sharing our toys: Cooperative learning versus collaborative learning. **Change**, pp. 13-18.

Chaffee, J. (Project director). (1989). **Thinking towards decisions** (Videotape). The critical thinking project/Annenberg/CPB project.

Chaffee, J. (1990). **Thinking critically** (3rd ed.). Boston: Houghton Mifflin.

Freiburger, O.A. (Fall/Spring 1995-1996). **Issues in nursing course manual**. Unpublished manuscript, Indiana University-Purdue University Fort Wayne at Fort Wayne, IN.

Johnson, D.W., Johnson, R.T., & Smith, K.A. (1991). **Active learning: Cooperation in the college classroom**. Edina, MN: Instruction Book Company.

Neuman, B. (1995). **The Neuman Systems Model** (3rd ed.). Norwalk CT: Appleton & Lange.

Chapter 8
Teaching Culturally Competent Care:
A Korean-American Experience
Nahn Joo Chang and Barbara T. Freese

The United States is increasingly recognizing and valuing the richness of its cultural heritage and population. Health care providers must be sensitive to cultural differences in order to provide effective care. For nursing, the essence of effective care is caring—among cultural and language differences.

As caring professionals, nurses must know clients as people of a culture in order to enable clients to improve health, face disability, or assist with dying (Leininger, 1991, p. 30). Nursing as caring is thus based on cultural sensitivity. The Council of Maori Nurses (New Zealand) describes nursing care that respects rather than violates the cultural beliefs and health practices of a given people as "culturally safe practice" (Watson, 1991, p. viii). This practice is based on understanding differences among dominant and divergent culture groups as well as differences between nurse and client. To develop this level of understanding, nurses must be able to conceptualize clients from their cultural perspective.

Betty Neuman emphasizes the importance of culture as the primary determinant of health belief systems and health behaviors. Neuman views culturally-determined values as central characteristics that comprise a client's core structure (Sohier, 1995, p. 102). In the Neuman nursing process format, nurses assess clients' perceptions of their condition in order to determine goals of care (Neuman, 1995, p. 37). This unique feature of the Neuman Systems Model promotes culturally sensitive care by incorporating explicit awareness of cultural differences into the nursing process.

Nurse educators are increasingly aware of the critical need to include culture content in curricula. Models that emphasize cultural sensitivity and diversity are useful in teaching these concepts to students. Before learning how to provide culturally competent care for clients of another culture, students must first become sensitive to the special needs of these clients.

The Cultural Variable

This chapter describes how a baccalaureate-level nursing program in rural South Carolina uses the expertise of a Korean-American faculty member to provide a learning experience based on the Neuman Systems Model (NSM) that sensitizes students to needs of people outside their own culture. In many ways the NSM provides an ideal framework to help students become sensitive to cultural differences and to incorporate this sensitivity into the care planning process.

First, the NSM conceptualizes the client system wholistically; the socio-cultural variable incorporates cultural factors into the students' understanding of clients. Second, the NSM focuses on an individual client as an integral part of the family system within its cultural context. This focus assists students to gain a full understanding of the importance of the family unit in other cultures and to become aware of the effects of stressors that threaten family system stability. Third, the Neuman nursing process format leads students to determine both client and caregiver perceptions for relevant goal setting. This unique characteristic of the model requires students to consider perceptual inconsistencies between nurse and client that result from cultural diversity along with those that result from individual differences.

Instructional Method

Caucasian and African-American are the two predominant cultures in rural South Carolina, with very few other cultures represented. Student populations in state-supported colleges and universities reflect this population mix. To introduce the concept of culturally competent care to classes composed of predominantly white and black learners, nursing students are provided a learning activity that includes a series of lecture-discussion sessions focused on a culturally unfamiliar population. The Korean-American population is selected because a Korean-American faculty member is available to provide a culturally-sensitive learning experience. The first session incorporates lecture material, a videotape that shows daily life in Korea, and a demonstration of Korean foods and practices—such as how to use chopsticks. Lively interaction with the Korean-American faculty member follows. Students are then guided through an instructional activity in which they use the NSM to analyze Korean-Americans and to identify nursing strategies that may be appropriate for dominant culture clients but could become stressors for this transcultural population. Finally, students prepare a brief report that is presented orally in class and submitted in written form for evaluation.

Prototype Class on Korean-American Families in the United States

Lecture. Korean-Americans are Koreans who have immigrated to the United States—many since the late 1960s. Approximately one million Korean-Americans in this country are striving for assimilation into American society while preserving and practicing Korean life patterns. They value being Korean and American simultaneously but are faced daily with language barriers and unfamiliar culture practices. These crosscultural stressors affect first generation Korean-Americans most strongly as they strive to lead a successful "dual life."

Korean-Americans may be viewed as communities of interest who share cultural values, beliefs, and life patterns. In metropolitan areas throughout the United States where such families live, there are supports to preserve Korean life patterns. These supports include Korean churches, shops, newspapers, language schools, and civic organizations. Korean churches play a major role in stress-reduction and problem-solving for these families as they provide for their spiritual, social, and educational needs. Families attend religious services and participate in recreational and supportive activities throughout the week. Most Korean-American congregations are Protestant Christian. Although Buddhism is the religion with the greatest number of followers in South Korea, it plays only a minor role for Korean-Americans.

Korean-American families. The family is valued much more highly in Korea than in America. The value accorded the family system represents one of the most important factors influencing life patterns in Korean-American society. As is true in Korea, Koreans in America are deeply committed to preserving the family system. A supreme obligation for any Korean is to preserve and enhance the prestige of his or her family. An informal but strict rule ensures the meeting of this obligation by all generations. Korean parents fulfill their obligation by sacrificing almost everything for the sake of their children. The parents exist in this world to provide the highest level of well-being possible for their children. In return, children are obliged to be obedient to their parents. Filial piety is thus the highest social norm in Korean society. This reciprocal relationship between parents and children remains the basic value for Koreans in America.

Health care. Cultural differences deeply affect Korean-Americans' access to health care and willingness to seek dominant-culture care providers. Because Koreans believe that Asian medicine such as ginseng and acupuncture helps promote health and prevent disease, this non-Western approach remains an important part of their health care. Korean-Americans purchase Asian herbal medicine supplies from Korean drug stores or directly from Korea. Non-Korean physicians and nurses often fail to provide culturally safe care because they do not understand the importance of including Asian medicine practices in the care provided. Consequently, Korean-American families are reluctant to seek care from health care providers of the dominant culture.

Another health care stressor for Korean-American families is arranging for care of dependent elderly relatives. In the Korean culture, it is the supreme obligation of children (especially of the eldest son) to provide for care of parents at home until their death (Chang and Chang, 1994). Because it is considered shameful for children to send their parents to nursing homes, Korean-American families are unable to accept the concept of elder care outside the home. Culturally competent care for these families must include measures to support the families in providing care within their homes.

Korean-Americans consult with Korean-American physicians in their community when health problems occur. For the physicians, these clients are an important segment of their clientele. Because these physicians understand Korean cultural values and speak the Korean language, Korean-American clients can seek health care from them without the added stress of communicating across language and culture barriers. By contrast, Korean-Americans who live in areas where no physicians of their culture practice experience extreme stress when they must seek health care from dominant-culture providers.

Concept application. Following the lecture-discussion on Korean-American families, students are instructed to work in small groups to analyze such a family as a client, using the information presented in class to respond to questions about culturally competent care. Students respond to Neuman concepts and questions about culturally competent care as shown in **Table 8.1.** The Neuman concepts are defined by students from a cultural perspective.

Table 8.1: Analysis of a Korean-American Family as Client

NSM Concepts	Student Responses (examples)
Central core	The family unit, including nuclear family and all generations, regardless of place of residence.
Lines of resistance	Inherited and shared cultural values and beliefs, e.g., the value placed on the family.
Normal line of defense	Korean language, strong extended family support.
Flexible line of defense	Involvement in Korean-American churches, organizations, and groups; access to Korean-American shops and restaurants; assistance from Korean-American experts (such as physicians and legal council).
Stressors (actual and potential)	Cultural shock, language barriers, and unfamiliar modes of health care management/delivery.
Primary prevention	Culturally appropriate health education through Korean-American organizations and churches.
Secondary prevention as intervention	Culturally safe interventions that accommodate different modes of treatment in American and Korean cultures and language barriers.
Tertiary prevention as intervention	Preventing recurrence of health problems following treatment by reinforcing treatment and health education at Korean-American group and church meetings or by a culturally safe provider.
Culture care questions	
Which stressors are most problematic for Korean-American families?	Language differences specific to English medical terms, differing modes of health care management, lack of support due to absence of family and friends, lack of interaction with non-Korean-Americans.
Describe how health care strategies that are appropriate in the dominant culture might become stressors for Korean-American families.	One example is the American norm of placing dependent elderly in nursing homes. Due to cultural differences, Korean-Americans consider it shameful to send their parents to a nursing home.

Evaluation of Outcomes

The effectiveness of this transcultural learning experience in sensitizing students to unique culturally-based client needs outside their own culture is evaluated using immediate and long-term outcome measures. The immediate outcome is the written report of the learning activity described previously, using the NSM to analyze families as clients. An example is provided in **Table 8.1**. The report is evaluated by faculty; feedback is given to students.

The long-term outcome will be evaluated by observing students giving culturally competent care to clients from diverse cultures. Emphasis on providing culturally sensitive care is continued as students plan care for clients in subsequent nursing courses. For example, in the community health nursing course, students usually encounter clients from cultures outside their own, including Hispanic- and African-American. Culturally sensitive care is promoted through use of client assessment and care planning based on the Neuman Nursing Process Format. Sensitivity to cultural differences enables students to be more effective in determining how client and caregiver perceptions differ, and how to accommodate these differences in setting relevant goals for divergent culture clients within their family systems.

Conclusion

Students must be sensitized to the unique needs of clients who are culturally different from themselves to establish the foundation for culturally competent care. The Neuman Systems Model provides a comprehensive framework for analysis of clients and families across cultures, from which appropriate nursing interventions can be based. An effective instructional approach involves providing students with information about other cultures through lecture-discussion by an individual of the culture followed by a guided analysis of that culture using the NSM. This approach enables the student to comprehend cultural differences and to distinguish dominant culture health care strategies that are appropriate from those that are not appropriate. The ultimate goal is to enable the student to provide culturally sensitive care to all clients.

References

Chang, C.S., & Chang, N.J. (1994). **The Korean management system: Cultural, political, economic foundations**. West Port, CT: Quorum Books.

Leininger, M.M. (1991). The theory of culture care diversity and universitality. In M.M. Leininger (Ed.), **Culture care diversity and universitality: A theory of nursing**, 5-72. New York: National League for Nursing.

Neuman, B. (1995). The Neuman Systems Model. In B. Neuman (Ed.), **The Neuman Systems Model** (3rd ed., pp. 3-44). Norwalk, CT: Appleton & Lange.

Sohier, R. (1995). Nursing care for the people of a small planet: Culture and the Neuman Systems Model. In B. Neuman (Ed.), **The Neuman Systems Model** (3rd ed., pp. 101-118). Norwalk, CT: Appleton & Lange.

Watson, J. (1991). Foreword. In M.M. Leininger (Ed.), **Culture care diversity and universitality: A theory of nursing**. New York: NLN Press.

Chapter 9
Community Health Nursing:
Keystone of Baccalaureate Education
Ann Weitzel and Kathryn Wood

A course in community health nursing is integral to all baccalaureate programs. It is one of the content areas that distinguishes baccalaureate education from associate degree and diploma programs. Community health courses afford students the opportunity to synthesize the knowledge and skills gained from other specialized content areas. Students practice critical thinking as they plan care, first for individuals, then families, and finally for communities.

At State University of New York (SUNY) Brockport, the Neuman Systems Model has provided the framework for both the presentation of theory and application to practice throughout the curriculum. The Neuman Systems Model (NSM) was selected after faculty reviewed several models and found that the propositions of Neuman's model were more congruent with their philosophy of Nursing. With the guidance of a consultant, the entire curriculum was redesigned from a Neuman perspective.

The culminating course in community health nursing enables students to synthesize concepts about clients as individuals and as members of families and then to focus on the community as "client." The course is composed of teaching modules and practice opportunities designed to meet needs of a diverse student population. This course affords flexibility for classroom teaching, self instruction, self pacing, and condensation of classroom materials so as to decrease in-class time. We have been able to offer the course as a directed study to a small group of students over the summer, meeting only one day a week for clinical experience and conferencing. We have offered the course at a community college a 2-hour drive from Brockport and condensed our classroom presentations to four or five sessions along with weekly clinical experiences to accommodate RN students seeking their baccalaureate degree. We have also offered the course in half-semester and full-semester blocks. Clinical experience is 1 day a week in a full-semester course and 2 days a week in a half-semester course. Six credits are given for completion of the course. The organization of the course, the independent learning that is possible, and the logic and adaptability of the Neuman model have enhanced the opportunity for collaboration and emphasis on critical thinking.

This methodology provides alternative ways to satisfy course objectives, allowing students to use their individual styles of learning and levels of ability. Students enjoy the opportunity to experiment, explore, and practice skills as many times as necessary and to be the center of the educational process. Benefits for the instructors include opportunity to increase the amount of personal contact with the student; easy updating of study materials because each module in the course is independent; and teaching and learning that can emphasize process rather than facts. These advantages also meet the goals of the new educational paradigm. This chapter addresses our approach to teaching both theory and practicum.

The course in community health nursing is organized into seven modules: The Community Health Nursing Role in a Home Health Agency; The Family as Client; Community Assessment; The Community as Client; Epidemiology: Applications in Community Health Nursing; Communicable Disease Control; Roles in Community Health Nursing.

The final module, Roles in Community Health Nursing, includes six minimodules: Community Health Nursing Role in a Home Health Agency: A Second Look; When the School is Client; Occupational Health Nursing; Discharge Planning; The Nurse as Health Planner; Forensic Nursing. Of these, two modules are required: Community Health Nursing Role in a Home Health Agency and Discharge Planning. Students work in teams, and every team must ensure that each of the optional modules is completed so that they can share their experiences.

The modular design has encouraged both self-paced learning and self-directed learning. The design has particular benefit for registered nurses who may have had some experience working in the community, which equips them to take tests for credit on content they know. We chose Cookfair's *Nursing Process and Practice in the Community* (1996) as our text because it presents most of the material for the course. Students also utilize additional resources that address family-centered nursing, communicable disease control, and national health goals. Over time, less emphasis has been placed on students pacing their own learning and more has been placed on providing opportunities for active learning and critical thinking.

Students are taught in the classroom how to perform family assessments. They are presented with case studies in which the diagnosis of an individual is presented. Students are challenged to infer the effects of the individual's problem on the family. Our original family assessment tool was modified to include a Neuman focus and organization based on Neuman's variables, using Berky and Hanson's (1991) adaptation, e.g., psychosocial, physical, developmental, and spiritual variables.

Reed's (1989) interpretation of the Neuman model assists students to identify specific family concepts and activities in each part of the model. For example, one of Reed's considerations is task allocation within the family, which she identifies as part of the flexible line of defense. In working with a family with an identified ill member, the task allocations are altered because the ill people cannot do what they are accustomed to doing. Students develop primary preventions to support the flexible line of defense, such as arranging for and supervising a home health aide to care for the ill family member and assisting the family in redistributing the family tasks. Students are helped to understand that these preventions keep a broad buffer between the flexible and normal lines of defense and maintain the family in a state of homeostasis or reconstitution at a different level.

Students also conduct community-assessment exercises in the classroom. This prepares them for conducting assessment of the actual community in the practicum component of the course. For this activity, students are divided into groups and given packets of information which provide a database for the community assessment and care plan for a homeless population. A tool previously developed by faculty to assess the community was modified to incorporate the model using the subsystems concepts described by Anderson and McFarlane (1988). An example of the use of this tool follows.

Community Health Practice

Community Health Nursing provides students an opportunity to explore the complexity of the community and apply theory to practice in the community setting. All levels of nursing intervention are particularly applicable in this environment and all levels of prevention are appropriate. As an example of primary prevention, students follow mother/child families identified from health department birth notices or referrals. They assist parents in anticipating potential problems such as childhood injuries and in preventing their occurrence. Occasionally, they are able to follow a family before and after the birth of a child. At the level of secondary prevention, students participate in blood pressure screening programs and in assessing and teaching clients receiving new medications or coping with the stress of new illness. For tertiary prevention, students supervise and teach home health aides to ensure the provision of high-quality rehabilitative care.

Our course provides multiple opportunities for collaboration with other health care professionals as students provide care in the home setting. Students work as part of the home health agency team, collaborating closely with primary nurses, attending physicians, physical therapists, social workers, and other support service personnel. The students function in case management and client advocate roles, as well as direct care. Students affiliate with one of several different agencies, including two county health department home health agencies—one a large urban agency and the other a small rural one. We also work with a large visiting nurse service which serves the same county as the urban health department. Each has advantages and disadvantages for our purposes. At the urban health department home health agency, students have the advantage of working in a sophisticated multidepartmental agency but because of its size and organization, may never appreciate it as a single agency. The small rural agency gives students an overview of suburban and rural health needs and the opportunity to see the whole agency functioning as a unit to meet those needs.

Student groups are assigned to one of the three agencies for their entire clinical rotation. Students meet together for class to share and learn from each other's experiences. We have recently begun to experiment with individual students having experience in both the urban and rural health departments. All students also have clinical experiences at a nonprofit community service agency located in the urban area. This agency distributes food, clothing, and other needed household items and offers health screenings and educational programs. Students participate in all aspects of this program.

Students care for clients and follow the rules of documentation for the specific agency. Clients come from several cultures, permitting assessment of Neuman's sociocultural variable in both the urban and rural settings. Students must function independently with families in the community, prioritizing problems and seeking guidance as needed. Although students are always under the supervision and guidance of a faculty member, the clinical experience encourages student autonomy because they are so often working independently with clients. Students are responsible for requesting updated orders, collaborating with various members of the health care team, and contacting the physician concerning the client's condition at home. Students also practice skills of group process. Working in teams, they schedule themselves to cover the group's joint responsibilities. This team approach fosters formation of leadership skills, creative problem solving, and cooperative group skills.

Students apply skills of family assessment in the clinical setting. Family assessment of clients includes consideration of cultural variables and their effect on nursing preventions. Students often select strong families who are suffering the temporary effects of the illness of one member. Some of the common problems addressed are communication issues, care for the caregiver, and the health of other family members. The family assessment and care plan are evaluated for a portion of the final grade.

Table 9.1 shows an example of what information is to be gathered and how it is to be organized. Following the data gathering, students summarize their information in terms of intra-, inter-, and extra-system stressors and identify family strengths. They categorize these strengths in terms of the family's perceptions and those of the care provider. Students list family nursing diagnoses and choose the three priorities for inclusion in the care plan. The care plan must be a realistic, working plan, including family goals and objectives, the dates these were negotiated with the family, preventions, family theory rationale for the preventions, family response, and modifications.

Table 9.2 shows a community assessment tool, which was adapted from Anderson and McFarlane's (1988) scheme of eight subsystems for the community. Those subsystems are physical environment, education, safety and transportation, politics and government, health and social services, communication, economics, and recreation. We refer to these subsystems as community variables, pointing out the comparison to and inclusion of the original Neuman variables in these subsystems. The physical variable is very evident in several of Anderson and McFarlane's (1988) subsystems. The psychological variable is most evident in education, health and social services, and communication. The sociocultural variable is included in the

Table 9.1: Family Assessment

I. Identifying Data
II. Description of Family (type of family, culture, race)
III. Characteristics of Housing
IV. Characteristics of Neighborhood
V. Genogram
VI. Possible Family Concerns, Concepts, and Interaction Patterns
    A. Psychosocial Relationship Characteristics
        1. Individual Family Member Needs
        2. Family and Individual Values
        3. Family Interaction Patterns
    B. Physical Status Characteristics
        1. Health Status of Individual Family Members
        2. Effect of Variances from Health on Family System
        3. Family's Health Care Knowledge and Attitudes
        4. Family's Life Style Patterns
        5. Family's Task Allocation to Carry Out Requirements and Responsibilities
        6. Family System's Balance (Point on Health-Illness Continuum)
    C. Developmental Characteristics
        1. Current Developmental Stage of Family
        2. Family's Ability to Complete Family Tasks
    D. Spiritual Characteristics
        1. Belief About Meaning of Life
        2. Purpose or Drive in Life
        3. Religious Affiliation
        4. Trust of Others
        5. Positive Sense of Self, Family, and Community
        6. Sense of Responsibility to Self, Family, and Community
        7. Feelings of Selflessness Among Family Members
        8. Ability to Love and be Loved
        9. Attitudes Toward Death/Losses

description of the core as well as education, politics, and government. The developmental variable is covered in the description of the core and in politics and government—which includes a history of the community. We have included the spiritual variable in the educational subsystem, where religious facilities and programs are listed.

Once students have completed the community assessment, they summarize it in terms of whether their client's stressors can be relieved and list the strongest and weakest variables within the community. Further, they identify the congruence of the community's perceptions of its strengths and stressors with their own. They formulate the community nursing diagnoses and categorize them as being intra-, inter-, or extra-system stressors. The care plan for the community nursing diagnosis includes community goals and objectives, preventions, a comparison to national health goals established in *Healthy People 2000* (1990), and an evaluation plan.

An example of a community care plan prepared by students addresses a finding of heart disease as a leading killer in a community where the predominant age group is between 29 and 35 and there are no exercise pro-

Table 9.2: Community Assessment

A. The Core
  1. Population Composition
  2. Population Characteristics (Include population origins, culture)
  3. Vital Statistics
B. Physical Environment
  1. Type of Community
  2. Geography
  3. Climate
  4. Housing
  5. Flora and Fauna
  6. Pollutants
  7. Animal Reservoirs or Vectors
C. Education
  1. Public and Private Educational Facilities
  2. Libraries
  3. Educational Services for Special Populations
  4. Religion/Spirituality
D. Safety and Transportation
  1. Public Safety Organizations
  2. Private Safety Organization
  3. Hazards
  4. Potential Hazards
  5. Emergency Medical System
  6. Transportation Resources
E. Politics and Government
  1. History of the Community
  2. Elected Leadership
  3. Non-official Leadership
  4. Accessibility of Leaders and Offices
  5. Neighborhood Mechanisms for Political Action
F. Health and Social Services
  1. Primary, Secondary, and Tertiary Health Care Sources
  2. Public and Private Welfare Resources
  3. Day Care Services
G. Communication
  1. Specific Resources
  2. Neighborhood Communication Resources
H. Economics
  1. Food Supply
  2. Major Industry and Business
  3. Banks, Savings and Loans, Credit Unions
  4. Shopping Areas
  5. Health Insurance
I. Recreation
  1. Public and Private Facilities
  2. Programs for Special Population Groups

grams available. The community's flexible line of defense is threatened and the community might establish a goal of increasing the physical activity of the population. This goal is consistent with *Healthy People 2000* goals to increase physical activity in order to decrease risk of cardiac disease. Preventions might include such things as working with the neighborhood association to locate funds and an appropriate site for offering exercise classes; locating a qualified person to present the exercise program; planning appropriate exercises to be taught; working with an agency nutritionist to offer dietary advice; finding an inexpensive printer to publish pamphlets and other needed materials for the program; publicizing the program, and recruiting participants.

The evaluation plan might include a pretest and posttest of participants to measure their change in physical activity. Preestablished goals for change would be set. This is a theoretical plan since there is not enough time in the semester for students to accomplish more than the assessment. However, it assists students in visualizing what could be accomplished in the community if time permitted. The use of *Healthy People 2000* helps the students to see what can be done in their community to work toward the achievement of national goals as well as introduces them to a valuable document for future reference.

Another unique aspect of our course is the emphasis on discharge planning. In addition to family and community assessments, students complete a discharge plan based on an observational experience. Each of our students spends a half day observing one of the discharge-planning nurses stationed at the local hospitals. These nurses are employed by the urban health department and visiting nurse services and are able to give our students an interesting look at discharge planning from a community health point of view. Students list assessment factors and stressors and submit a referral form complete with skilled nursing orders. They identify ways for the discharge planning nurse to evaluate the plan and determine whether it was successful. Students frequently comment that they did not know discharge planning nurses were available in the hospital and certainly have a much better idea of how to write a community health referral after this experience.

The above activities are required of every student. As indicated previously, students also choose one of these four optional modules for further experience: school nursing, occupational health nursing, health planning, or forensic nursing. For implementing the health planning module, our college has the good fortune to be located near Rochester, New York, which is widely known for its legacy of community health planning. We have introduced the students to the local health systems agency by taking them to meetings where decisions are being made about construction of new facilities, expansion of existing facilities, and adding services where they do not presently exist. One of our faculty members is active with the health systems agency so students can see nurses functioning in a somewhat different—and expanded—role.

Conclusion

It seems we might have found the perfect match of model to curriculum. The Neuman Systems Model has strengthened our curriculum by giving us the matrix we needed to hold concepts and theories together. Faculty have found the model easy to use and live with as we continue to refine the curriculum. Students have reacted positively to the model as well. It seems to give order to a challenging curriculum.

Faculty continue to explore the Neuman Systems Model and apply it to their own practice and teaching. The model gives structure but allows flexibility. Faculty are able to examine their own views and interpretation of the model and share their insights with fellow faculty. In this manner the curriculum continues to be enriched. Community Health Nursing has certainly been strengthened by incorporating the Neuman Systems Model. The logic and adaptability of the model for all categories of clients have made the course flexible and adaptable to a variety of learning situations.

References

Anderson, E.T., & McFarlane, J.M. (1988). **Community as Client: Application of the Nursing Process**. Philadelphia: J.B. Lippincott.

Berky, K.M., & Hanson, S.M. (1991). **Family Assessment and Interventions**. St. Louis: Mosby.

Cookfair, M.M. (1996). **Nursing Care in the Community**. St. Louis: Mosby.

Reed, K.S. (1989). Family Theory Related to the Neuman Systems Model. In B. Neuman (Ed.), **The Neuman Systems Model** (2nd ed., pp. 385-395). Norwalk, CT: Appleton & Lange.

U.S. Public Health Service. (1990). **Healthy People 2000: National Health Promotions and Disease Preventions Objectives**. (DHHS Publication No. (PHS) 91-50213). Washington, DC: U.S. Government Printing Office.

Chapter 10
Primary Prevention in an Associate of Science Curriculum
Rita Sutherland and Donna L. Forrest

Primary prevention is a concept whose time has come. Insurance providers are providing third-party reimbursement for preventive health care to curb increasing health care costs. Nurses are recognized as the professionals who provide primary prevention through teaching clients to attain, maintain, and retain health. These facts lead nurse educators to design curricula that emphasize health promotion and disease prevention as a direct response to societal needs. This chapter describes a unique Associate of Science Curriculum, which emphasizes primary prevention.

Primary Prevention Strategies

The Santa Fe Community College (SFCC) nursing faculty believe that primary prevention should be a theme throughout all nursing intervention courses in the curriculum. After a thorough search for a health care model that best suited this philosophy, faculty selected The Neuman Systems Model (NSM) as a guide for the curriculum structure. Three nursing programs at SFCC are based on this model: the 2-year Associate of Science Degree in Nursing (ASN), the ASN Bridge Program (LPN to ASN), and the Practical Nurse Program (PN).

The Neuman Systems Model emphasizes primary prevention principles in all three modes of intervention—primary, secondary, and tertiary. According to Neuman (1982) primary prevention is appropriate when there is some "risk or hazard" present in an individual's internal or external environment. This risk is a stressor that threatens to break through the person's lines of defense causing some degree of reaction. When this potential is present, Neuman (1995) states that nursing intervention is aimed at reducing the possibility of client encounter with stressors and strengthening the client's flexible line of defense so stability of the client system is maintained. These propositions of NSM guide faculty to assist students in recognizing and coping with stressors in their own lives and the lives of the clients they serve.

Faculty commitment to use of primary prevention in every mode of nursing intervention is evidenced by the inclusion of primary prevention objectives in each Nursing Process syllabus. Each area of study follows a common course outline that includes nursing roles, nursing process, and nursing knowledge. Primary prevention interventions are taught within the nursing process format. Assessment of populations at risk helps students to identify clients who are in need of primary prevention measures. Primary prevention interventions include ways to strengthen clients' lines of defense and reduce stressors through teaching, counseling, identifying client strengths, and support systems.

Table 10.1: Nursing Process I: Self-Awareness Classroom Exercise

The Neuman Systems Model offers a new way of thinking, a systematic way to organize the material you are receiving now in NP-I and the material you will receive as you move through the following nursing processes.

It even offers a way for you to gain self-awareness and look at your own development as a student nurse, graduate nurse, and nurse practitioner. You can use the "five human variables" to examine the stressors in your own life and how you react to them. This exercise in self-awareness will help you to understand "the therapeutic use of self."

DIRECTIONS

Gather into small groups of 5 or 6 students. Use Neuman Systems Model to assess:
1. Current stressors in your life.
2. The strength/weakness of your:
    a.   flexible lines of defense
    b.   normal lines of defense
    c.   lines of resistance
    d.   core (related to specific core needs)
3. Your place on the health/illness continuum
4. Your level of development

Select one person to be "reporter" who will relate the findings back to the class. (The person reporting does not have to be the one whose life is assessed.)

In the first of five Nursing Process courses (NP-I) four exercises are introduced to help the students understand the fundamental concepts of the model. In the first exercise, students are divided into groups of five or six and are asked to identify and discuss actual and potential stressors in their own lives. Next, they are instructed to assess the strengths of their own flexible and normal lines of defense (**Table 10.1**). As self-awareness grows, students quickly learn that many of their individual concerns are shared by others in the group.

In a subsequent class, students complete the Holmes and Masuda Life Crisis Scale (Wilson & Kneisl, 1991) and contract to make a specific change in their own lives. This exercise illustrates the principles of reducing the intensity and duration of stressors and strengthening flexible lines of defense. The contract emphasizes one change students can make that will help them evolve toward a wellness lifestyle. Emphasis is on areas that have an immediate strengthening effect on the flexible line of defense or ways to diminish stressors, such as better eating habits, cessation of smoking, and adopting a regular exercise routine. **Table 10.2** shows a student personal self-care plan.

A second exercise, introduced in the first semester of the nursing process courses, provides an opportunity for developing self-awareness on specific nursing-related topics. Students meet in groups of 10-12 for a 2-hour session each week for 8 weeks. With the guidance of a faculty group leader,

students explore their values, attitudes, and feelings ɪ
tionships, grief and loss, assertiveness, sexuality, prof€
areas of interest and concern. The group experience
ate self disclosure and opportunities to learn grou'
examination is a beginning for the movement from ɪ
Benner (1984) has noted from conversations with nuɪɔɪ..ɡ
said it was important for them to come to terms in some personal way w ɪ..
what the patient was confronting before they became good at working with
patients with particular illnesses" (Benner p. 165). The emphasis on primary prevention in the students' lives sets the foundation for students to
transfer this knowledge when providing client care.

Often the focus of primary prevention is to actively listen to clients' needs
or concerns and provide clarification, feedback, or information in return.
Teaching facilitative communication skills is a challenge for educators. Didactic material is necessary but, as is true of all skills, practice is the key to
effective mastery. In the nursing process courses, students complete a Therapeutic Communication Exercise involving audio taping a client of their choice
30 minutes per week for 6 weeks. In groups of three or four students they
listen to their tapes and discuss with a faculty member the communication
process as they observe it evolving. Prior to each of these discussions students have reviewed the tapes and identified various communication tech-

---

Table 10.2: Nursing Process I: Worksheet for Developing a Personal Self-Care Plan

My main area of interest (eating, exercise, learning to deal with common illness problems, etc.):

My main personal strengths and resources in this area:

The best resources for me in this area (people, groups, classes, etc.):

Some activities and goals I might choose to help me explore this area (Brainstorm):

I would like to choose an initial activity that I could complete in about ___days/weeks/ months.

Within this time limit, the goal I'd most like to set for myself is:

Some small rewards I will give myself for making progress toward this goal:

A big reward I will give myself for reaching my goal:

I will ask _____ to be my support person in working toward this goal.

I will contact my support person on _____ (date) to bring him/her up to date on my exploration in this area.

My Commitment, again, is to accomplish the following activities:

between now and the following date:

On that date I will give my support person a report on my explorations in this area.

_____   _____
Signature   Today's Date

used. They are instructed to begin the first session with their client by
ng, "Tell me about one of your concerns." This helps elicit the stressors
e client is experiencing. Later in the process, students ask their clients to
look at alternative behaviors that would strengthen the client's ability to cope
with stressors–ways in which they can diminish the stressors in their lives or
strengthen their lines of defense to decrease the negative effect of stressors.
These four learning activities accomplished in the first semester of the nursing
program undergird students' understanding of primary prevention as a nursing intervention.

During the first semester, students are also introduced to alternative healing
methods such as massage, reflexology, and acupuncture. Therapeutic touch is
demonstrated and students are given the opportunity to practice this skill with
other students as clients. Basic nursing skills and practices are also taught,
including universal precautions, assisting clients with hygiene and other activities of daily living, transferring and moving clients, range of motion exercises, medical and surgical asepsis, and assessing vital signs.

Primary prevention continues to be emphasized in the following four semesters. **Tables 10.3** and **10.4** show examples of how the common course
outline is used to ensure continuity when teaching very different content areas; e.g., a client with psycho-physiologic problems (**Table 10.3**) and one with
circulation and respiratory problems (**Table 10.4**). Students soon discover that
primary prevention is necessary at each level of intervention and at each stage
of life-span development.

In caring for mothers and infants in NP-IV, students learn that prenatal care
enhances the likelihood of a normal delivery and a healthy baby. They see that
Lamaze training and parenting classes help both mothers and fathers to bond
to one another and to the new child, strengthening family ties and commitment. In caring for well children, students learn the effectiveness of immunizations. Students are also required to complete a teaching project with small
children. In groups of six or seven, students select, plan, organize, and give a
15- to 30-minute presentation on a wellness subject.

For example, six students in their fourth semester presented a class on hand
washing for 4 and 5 year olds at a preschool nursery. This project included a 4-
minute video segment of Snow White telling the seven dwarfs why they must
wash their hands before eating. By shaking hands and touching their faces,
the nursing students passed "germs" in the form of colored stickers from one
to another. The children passed "germs" to one another, only this time the
germs were dry oatmeal in peanut butter. After a hilarious but controlled pass-
ing of "germs," the children were each taken to the sink and instructed in
effective hand washing. This was followed by a lively discussion underscoring
the lesson and giving the nursing students a chance to evaluate the effectiveness of their presentation.

At every stage of development, assessment of specific populations at risk is
required. For example while caring for clients in acute care settings, students
are required to complete Nursing Process Records (NPRs). Under the heading

**Table 10.3: Application of Common Course Outline
Nursing Process II
Care of the Client with Psycho-physiological Illness**

In teaching about the core need anxiety, Care of the Client with Psycho-physiological Illness, the following content is found under Planning, Implementing, and Evaluating Care:

I. **PRIMARY PREVENTION**
    A. ASSESSMENT
        1. *Population at risk*
            a. personality types
            b. characteristics
                (1) pessimistic
                (2) helplessness
                (3) hopelessness
                (4) depression
                (5) inability to express emotions
        2. *Secondary gains*
        3. *Clients' perception of stressors*

    B. INTERVENTION
        1. *Positive self-talk*
            a. thought stopping
            b. power language
        2. *Time management*
            a. make "to do" list
            b. prioritize tasks
            c. accept that all cannot be done
            d. plan to do disliked tasks when energy is high
            e. plan enjoyable tasks when energy is at it's lowest ebb
            f. delegate
        3. *Social support*
        4. *Decrease stressors*
            a. negative emotions
                (1) guilt
                (2) anger
            b. use humor to combat negative thinking and feeling

"Nursing Orders" in the NPR, students must address primary, secondary, and tertiary prevention strategies. In the fifth and final semester of the program, students work with mentally ill clients in a tertiary setting. In this setting, primary prevention strategies of teaching and counseling are vital. Students complete a Communication Process Record with their clients concerning such subjects as medications.

Additionally, a term paper addressing "Health Problems Affecting Behavior" is required. Each student defines the mental disorder diagnosis of a client and gives information related to the classification and types of the disorder, theories of etiology, incidence, and population at risk. Students identify areas where primary prevention should take place in the section on etiology, incidence,

**Table 10.4: Application of Common Course Outline
Nursing Process IV
Care of the Client with Circulation and Aeration Needs**

The common course outline is also used to teach Circulation and Aeration: Caring for the Client with Atherosclerosis.

Planning, Implementing, and Evaluating Care:

I. **PRIMARY PREVENTION**
    A. ASSESS THE POPULATION AT RISK USING THE AMERICAN HEART ASSOCIATION'S RISKS INCLUDING:
        1. age (elderly)
        2. cigarette smoking
        3. emotional stress
        4. hyperlipidemia
        5. gender (male)
        6. hypertension
        7. diabetes mellitus
        8. obesity
        9. lack of exercise
        10. family history

    B.INTERVENTION
        1. take a health history
        2. plan risk reduction
        3. teaching and counseling

and population at risk. Students are instructed to assess for stressors and potential stressors that may affect the five variables and lines of defense wholistically. Finally, the students incorporate their findings in determining the necessary nursing actions in each mode of intervention: primary, secondary, and tertiary as shown in **Table 10.5**.

As students move into clients' homes to give care, they will continue to assess health status, stressors, and lines of defense for both the client and the environment. Students are expected to plan care using all modes of intervention and are evaluated in all semesters for their use of primary prevention interventions.

Perceptions of Curriculum

Students demonstrate that they value primary prevention in a variety of ways. One student surveyed a group of 15 clients who had recently been transferred from a critical care unit (CCU) to a step-down unit. She asked, "What, in your opinion was the most important service rendered by the nurses in CCU?" Four choices were given as possible answers (a) close monitoring, (b) provided medically ordered interventions—treatments and medications, (c) called me by name, and (d)explained procedures and how I was progressing. Fifty percent of the clients chose the fourth option. This response confirmed the student's hypothesis that the primary prevention strategies of teaching and facilitative communication are necessary to reduce clients' levels of anxiety in high-tech critical care areas.

Another example of how students perceive the importance of primary prevention occurred in a spontaneous, non-solicited fashion. After spending 3 weeks in a rehabilitation center caring for stroke and spinal cord injured clients, students were asked to write a critique of the clinical site with special emphasis on how they perceived the role of the registered nurse in this tertiary setting. Faculty did not specifically require students to address modes of prevention in the critique. Thus, it came as a welcome surprise to learn that students mentioned primary prevention strategies *as the*

**Table 10.5: Application of Common Course Outline
Nursing Process V
Health Problems Affecting Client Behavior: Paper Guidelines**

I. MUST BE PRESENTED IN COLLEGE RESEARCH PAPER FORM
    A. LEGIBLE (2 pts)
    B. GRAMMATICALLY CORRECT (2 pts)
    C. REFERENCES AND BIBLIOGRAPHY INCLUDED IN APA STYLE (2 pts)
    D. INTEGRATION OF CONCEPTS (5 pts)
    E. LIMIT TO 10 - 12 TYPED PAGES

II. INCLUDE IN THE BODY OF THE PAPER
    A. DETAILED DESCRIPTION OF DISORDER
        1. Definition of the mental disorder (4 pts)
        2. Classification/type (4 pts)
        3. Theories of etiology (4 pts)
        4. Incidence/populational risk (4 pts)
    B. CLIENT ASSESSMENT
        1. Precipitating stressors and effect upon normal and flexible lines of defense (10 pts)
        2. Degrees of reaction (typical behaviors). Asterisk client's signs and symptoms (10 pts)
        3. A nursing diagnosis which is a statement of the relationship of disorder to anxiety (4 pts)
        4. Wholistic effect on human variables of client
            a. Psychological (5 pts)
            b. Physiological (5 pts)
            c. Sociocultural (5 pts)
            d. Developmental (5 pts)
            e. Spiritual (5 pts)
    C. HIGH RISK AND ACTUAL NURSING DIAGNOSES FOR CLIENT FROM NANDA LIST. MUST HAVE AT LEAST 10 NURSING DIAGNOSES (10 pts)
    D. SPECIFIC NURSING ORDERS FOR THREE OF THE NURSING DIAGNOSES LISTED ABOVE (10 pts)
        1. There must be at least five orders for each of the nursing diagnoses.
        2. Must include at least one nursing order for each mode of prevention (primary, secondary, and tertiary).

---

most important nursing actions. The most important role, they agreed, was teaching. Another frequently stated primary prevention strategy was proper use of transfer techniques to ensure safety for both clients and caretakers. Other skills emphasized were facilitative communication, nurses' assertiveness on behalf of clients' welfare, and proper use of restraints.

Interviews of new graduates revealed that they were equally committed to the use of primary prevention. This was an expected response coming from a graduate practicing in the Alachua County Public Heath Center. He stated that nearly all his nursing actions were preventive: teaching, counseling, and giving immunizations primarily. Graduates in a variety of other areas also voiced commitment to the use of primary prevention strategies. A recent graduate working in a psychiatric hospital stated that primary prevention was a major focus for him. He was especially concerned about clients' lack of compliance with medication regimes. "The only method of dealing with the problem short of force," he said, "is teaching, teaching, teaching!" A graduate working in a step-down unit for cardiac clients expressed discomfort at not having enough time to do all the primary preventive measures she would like. Nevertheless, she takes time between and during task-focused care to explain to her clients what is happening in terms of their treatments and procedures and to teach them about cardiac risk factors and medications. She also cited teaching activities during discharge planning as an important primary prevention strategy. All of the graduate nurses contacted valued primary prevention as a nursing intervention and felt rewarded when clients responded with beneficial changes in behaviors.

Tabulation of results of the annual Graduate Students' Survey in 1994 shows that 98% of SFCC graduates reported using primary prevention strategies in promoting clients' optimal level of health and preventing illness. Ninety-eight percent of graduating students reported they include health counseling and discharge teaching in the development of clients' care plans, and 94% implement teaching and/or discharge planning specific to the clients' level of development, knowledge, and learning needs. Further, 93% of the students agreed that the learning experiences and methods of instruction used in the SFCC ASN Program helped them fulfill the educational outcomes required for each nursing course. Implicit in the survey responses are (a) primary prevention strategies are valued as necessary nursing actions and (b) the experiences and instruction of their courses prepared them to use primary prevention in their nursing practice. As noted by Benner (1984) students are taught about nursing situations in terms of "objective attributes," that is, using concrete instructions for beginning skills development. It is not surprising then, when asked about their use of primary prevention in clinical areas, both students and new graduates responded with examples of specific nursing skills such as teaching, counseling, immunizations, and the use of safety measures such as hand washing, putting up side rails, and using universal precautions.

Faculty were more likely than students to comment on the broader effects of teaching primary prevention in a primary health care market. One faculty member stated that primary prevention is an "excellent way to save money in health care since 70% of hospital admissions are due to chronic diseases that could have been prevented by healthier lifestyles." Faculty use primary prevention as an opportunity to emphasize "healthy living." As one faculty member said, "Incidental teaching comes up all the time if one views his/her role as an informer for health care." There is consensus among SFCC nursing faculty and students that primary prevention must be a major focus of practicing nurses, especially in the current health care system. We have a professional imperative to lead in this movement to promote the health and well-being of all people.

References

Benner, P. (1984). **From Novice to Expert: Excellence and Power in Clinical Nursing Practice**. Menlo Park, CA: Addison-Wesley.

Neuman, B. (1995). **The Neuman Systems Model** (3 ed.). Norwalk, CT: Appleton & Lange.

Neuman, B. (1982). **The Neuman Systems Model: Application to Nursing Education and Practice**. Norwalk, CT: Appleton-Century-Crofts.

Wilson, H., & Kneisl, C. (1991). **Psychological Nursing Concepts: An Activity Book**. New York: Addison-Wesley.

Chapter 11
The Neuman Systems Model in Advanced Practice Nursing
Patricia Nuttall, Eleanor M. Stittich, and Filomena C. Flores

Rapid change in the delivery and financing of health care has led the nursing profession to develop an agenda for health care reform that promotes cost-effective, high-quality care for all consumers. The health care reform agenda prompted nurse educators to redesign master's level curricula to prepare advanced practice nurses (APN) for collaborative and autonomous practice. Master's degree curricula must include the essentials recommended by the American Association of Colleges of Nursing (AACN, 1995) as well as the six domains recommended by the National Organization of Nurse Practitioner Faculties (NONPF, 1995). Graduates of curricula that meet these requirements are then eligible for national certification examinations. The depth and breadth of knowledge required by advanced practice nurses challenges educators to design curricula that promote syntactical and inquiry learning. Thus, the goal of master's education is to prepare professionals as scholar-clinicians who incorporate theory, research findings, and supportive scientific rationale in their clinical practice.

The Nurse Practitioner Program at California State University, Fresno
The purpose of the program at California State University, Fresno (CSUF) is to prepare nurse practitioners who are specialists in interdisciplinary case management and who offer high-quality, culturally sensitive primary health and nursing care to clients in community-based and ambulatory care settings (CSUF, 1995). The program is committed to preparing nurse practitioners who will provide increased availability of health care services in response to a wide range of health problems of clients, families, and communities. The advanced practice nurse program prepares its graduates as family nurse practitioners, pediatric nurse practitioners, and school nurse/pediatric nurse practitioners. New tracks for the geriatric nurse practitioner and community health clinical nurse specialist are also in the planning stages.

An underlying goal of this program is to recruit and retain students who reflect the diversity of the clients they serve and are interested in practicing in underserved rural and urban communities with at-risk client populations. At the present time, California is in the midst of unparalleled demographic change, as reflected in dramatic increases in minority, refugee, immigrant, and economically disadvantaged populations. In particular, the Hispanic and Southeast Asian population is increasing markedly because of immigration and high birthrates. California also has a high percentage of aging citizens. The increased growth rate, coupled with the shortage and poor distribution of family practice physicians and a scarcity of existing primary care services in California have intensified the need for the primary care services of qualified nurse practitioners.

The Neuman Systems Model (NSM) is used as a guiding framework for curriculum organization, sequencing of courses, and evaluation of learning. The wholistic view of the model sets the standard for the preparation of nurse practitioners who are capable of delivering direct, expert primary care services to a diverse population of consumers. The particular strength of the NSM for the nurse practitioner program lies in its organization of content related to the delivery of care to clients across the health continuum within the levels of primary, secondary, and tertiary prevention. A cross-cultural perspective at all three levels of prevention helps students learn how to consider cultural diversity in a variety of systems. They learn how to effectively plan health assessment, health maintenance, and health promotion for optimal client wellness (Stittich, Flores, & Nuttall, 1995).

NSM propositions encourage client involvement and participation in health care. This is particularly important for the advanced nurse practitioner when helping the client assume more responsibility for self-care as well as for selection of appropriate providers. Addition to the model of the "created environment" concept helps nurses to be knowledgeable in ways that facilitate clients in modifying their state of wellness. This component "represents the client's unconscious mobilization of all system variables toward system stability and integrity ... and is inherently purposeful and functions as a protective shield or safe arena for the system" (Breckenridge, 1992, p. 2). The nurse practitioner must continue to give preventive care and include health teaching to educate consumers on essential aspects of healthful living habits and practices. Hence, the wholistic perspective in the Neuman Model (physiological, psychological, sociocultural, developmental, and spiritual) provides all essential components for the nurse practitioner program. This wholism gives the NSM a key advantage for selecting and guiding teaching and learning in advanced practice nursing.

The Teaching-Learning Process in the Nurse Practitioner Program
The systematic framework of the Neuman Systems Model facilitates teaching of core concepts of systematic inquiry, advanced practice, and social organization essential for independent practice (Stittich, Avent, & Patterson 1989). Teaching and learning in the nurse practitioner curriculum is based on a paradigm that emphasizes critical thinking and contextual and syntactical learning. A main advantage of the Neuman-based curriculum at the graduate level is its utility as a guiding framework for the development of strong clinical judgment skills in the diagnosis and management for nursing and general health care needs of clients.

Boyd (1992) describes the teaching process as a planned and purposeful activity that assures learning. The Neuman model provides the plan for the practitioner student to assess the physiologic, psychologic, sociocultural, developmental, and spiritual variables of the client, the types of stressors prevailing in the internal and external milieu of the individual, the responses to these stressors, and appropriate nursing interventions. Complete assessment of the client requires substantial recognition of all intra-, inter-, and extra-personal stressors.

An assessment of each person's coping patterns adds to an understanding of the ways a person deals with stress. This database enables the nurse practitioner to guide clients in using their resources to return to a steady state of balance or stable state of wellness. The educational methods used for courses in the nurse practitioner program advocate self-direction, critical thinking, and inquiry learning. Students are active participants in their learning. The courses on primary, secondary, and tertiary preventions as interventions include opportunities for experiential learning.

Colgrove, Schlapman, and Erpelding (1996) define experiential learning as an approach that focuses on the role of experience in learning. This process of learning considers reflection as a main channel in the transformation of knowledge from information to new meanings and ideas. Students reflect on personal experiences, discuss thoughts and observations with others, and reevaluate what is known and understood. This interaction, discussion, and reevaluation lead to improved comprehension and interpretation of the learning experiences.

Colgrove and colleagues (1996) also describe the merits of experiential learning as process orientation, wholism, person and environment focus, and resolution of conflicts between concrete experiences and abstract concepts. Students, therefore, become directly involved in the active process of learning.

Nurse practitioners should develop ingenuity, initiative, and resourcefulness for their own learning. Teaching strategies are selected to stimulate student involvement in discussions and independent study. The instructional methods used in theory courses to cultivate creativity and increase learning include seminar-discussion, role-playing, simulations, problem-solving exercises, instructional media, and autotutorial and structured learning activities. Clinical courses include a preceptor-supervised practicum in clinics, health maintenance organizations (HMOs), health agencies, schools, physicians' offices, and other health care settings. Other examples of teaching learning approaches are student-faculty-preceptor conferences, clinical seminars, case management studies, grand rounds, student-prepared patient educational tools, and presentations.

The multidisciplinary and multicultural backgrounds of the students and multicultural backgrounds of the clients serve as valuable resources for enhancement of learning for subsequent practice. A common thread in all teaching is the emphasis on collaboration involving respect for, and ability to work with, other health care providers in meeting client goals. This strategy capitalizes on the growing trend toward a more collegial and complementary relationship among physicians, nurses, and other health care providers (Rankin & Stallings, 1990).

The preceptorial experience of the faculty member enables the student to work with clinical experts in specific health care agencies. Lambert,

McDonough, Pond, and Billue (1996) emphasize that this strategy allows the student to socialize with experts while developing their role as nurse practitioners. It also gives the students opportunity for independent problem solving. The role models are unit-based care givers who engage in one-to-one teaching experiences with the nurse practitioner student while actively involved in patient care. This experience promotes realistic learning and facilitates transition into practice upon completion of the program.

According to Fuszard and Taylor (1996), preceptors and students establish a special "mentor-protégé" relationship. The mentors are carefully selected: all demonstrate successful performance in their practice, with willingness and ability to assume the responsibility of teaching, guiding, and supervising nurse practitioner students in the clinical setting. While the preceptors and the faculty work cooperatively in the selection and guidance of clinical experiences, the faculty assist the preceptors in understanding and implementing clinical learning within the Neuman Systems Model framework. Students are guided in the integration of these concepts with nursing, role, and family theories in their clinical practice. Students' achievement of this process is subsequently depicted in clinical performance, simulation exercises, seminars, classroom discussions of clinical experiences, and ability of students to move into the advanced practice nursing role.

Descriptions of the nurse practitioner program (Stittich et al., 1995) and the pediatric and family nurse practitioner programs (Stittich et al., 1995) are included in *The Neuman Systems Model* (1989 and 1995). At CSUF, the first year of the program contains core content required by all students, including theoretical foundations. Although the NSM is the organizational framework for the curriculum, other theories are also introduced. A key teaching strategy for this course is to critique and analyze extant nursing theories and to determine the relationship between theory and research. Through the teaching strategies students learn the value and use of nursing theory in clinical practice. Throughout four consecutive semesters students focus on interventions for primary, secondary, and tertiary preventions as well as pharmacologic and non-pharmacologic approaches to client management. Student learning includes the selection of appropriate management modalities based on established protocols or algorithms, potential risk, cost containment, and client acceptability.

Outcomes of Advanced Practice Nurse Curriculum

Nursing outcomes are monitored by evaluating specific nursing interventions used in one or more of the prevention modes (Neuman, 1995). The successful use of the NSM in the nurse practitioner program is evident in the ability of graduates to meet the wholistic needs of the clients and families in their care.

Several methods of evaluation are used to determine terminal competencies. These include periodic informal feedback and questionnaire data collection from employers of graduates of the program and exit interviews with graduates upon their completion of the program. Students also receive evaluations each semester at midterm and at the completion of each clinical practicum; and preceptors are encouraged to submit a written annual program and experience evaluation.

During faculty telephone conferences and visits to clinical sites, informal feedback from preceptors is received relevant to individual student performance and total program offerings. A detailed student evaluation tool for use at exit from the program is in the developmental stage. Development and refinement of program evaluation tools continue. One of the most satisfactory methods of evaluation is networking with the large number of students who are employed in the central valley. Virtually all graduates of the program are employed as nurse practitioners upon graduation.

In summary, the nurse-practitioner program at CSUF synthesizes the role of the nurses in advanced practice nursing in primary, secondary, and tertiary care. The breadth of the NSM, the client focus, emphasis on primary prevention, and coordinated managed care confirm its effectiveness as a framework for advanced practice nursing (Lowry, Walker, & Mirenda, 1995). It serves as a complete framework for the assessment, diagnosis, planning, intervention, and evaluation of nursing measures in meeting health care needs of clients in primary care settings. Implications for further usefulness will be evident through continued application, study, and research in advanced practice nursing.

References

AACN. (1995). **Essentials of master's education for advanced practice nursing**. Washington, DC: American Association of Colleges of Nursing.

Breckenridge, D. (1992, March). A brief update on the Neuman systems model. **Neuman News. 3(1)**, 2.

Boyd, M. (1992). The teaching process. In N. Whitman, B. Graham, C. Gleit, and M. Boyd (Eds.), **Teaching in nursing practice: A professional model** (pp. 155-172). Norwalk, CT: Appleton & Lange.

California State University, Fresno. (1995). **General catalog 1995-1996**. Fresno, CA: California State University, Fresno.

Colgrove, S., Schlapman, N., & Erpelding, C. (1996). Experiential Learning. In B. Fuszard (Ed.), **Innovative teaching strategies in nursing** (pp. 9-17). Gaithersburg, MD: Aspen.

Fuszard, B., & Taylor, L. (1996). Mentorship. In B. Fuszard (Ed.), **Innovative teaching strategies in nursing** (pp. 200-208). Gaithersburg, MD: Aspen.

Lambert, V., McDonough, J., Pond, E., & Billue, J. (1996). Preceptorial experience. In B. Fuszard (Ed.), **Innovative teaching strategies in nursing** (pp. 191-194). Gaithersburg, MD: Aspen.

Lowry, L., Walker, P., & Mirenda, R. (1995). Through the looking glass: Back to the future. In B. Neuman (Ed.), **The Neuman Systems Model** (3rd ed., pp. 63-76). Norwalk, CT: Appleton & Lange.

National Organization of Nurse Practitioner Faculties. (1995). **Advanced nursing practice: Curriculum guidelines and program standards for nurse practitioner education**. Washington, DC: National Organization of Nurse Practitioner Faculties.

Neuman, B. (1989). **The Neuman Systems Model** (2nd ed.). Norwalk, CT: Appleton & Lange.

Neuman, B. (1995). **The Neuman Systems Model** (3rd ed.). Norwalk, CT: Appleton & Lange.

Rankin, S., & Stallings, K. (1990). **Patient education: Issues, principles, & practices**. Philadelphia: Lippincott.

Stittich, E., Avent, C., & Patterson, K. (1989). Neuman-based baccalaureate and graduate nursing programs, CSUF. In B. Neuman (Ed.), **The Neuman Systems Model** (2nd ed., pp. 163-174). Norwalk, CT: Appleton & Lange.

Stittich, E., Flores, F., & Nuttall, P. (1995). Cultural considerations in a Neuman-based curriculum. In B. Neuman, (Ed.), **The Neuman Systems Model** (3rd ed., pp. 147-162). Norwalk, CT: Appleton & Lange.

Unit III: Outcomes, Opportunities, and Challenges

"Seeing is Believing.
I wouldn't have seen it if I had not believed it."
—Anonymous

Evaluators examine and judge the value and worth of the object under evaluation. Processes of educational evaluation have traditionally reflected the behaviorist approach. Evaluation tools, however, often become the focus within the nursing education process. As educational processes reflect a more humane approach, so must evaluation methods demonstrate a cooperative activity between students and faculty. Thus the effects of the curriculum on students can be better determined. Chapters in Unit III describe program evaluation processes and final outcomes that demonstrate the efficacy of the Neuman Systems Model as a framework for nursing education.

Chapter 12
Fourth-Generation Evaluation and the Neuman Systems Model
Bronwynne Evans

"Evaluation carried out properly in an environment of trust and respect between teacher and learner aids both the teacher in the instructional process and the student in the learning process" (Reilly & Oermann, 1992, p. 380). Why, then, is evaluation so dreaded by nursing students and faculty alike? Why does the formal evaluation of clinical competency diminish rather than foster the atmosphere of trust and cooperative learning so highly valued by today's nursing instructors? How can today's caring faculty continue to use the adversarial process of evaluation? This chapter will present the approach of a Neuman-based associate degree program to these important questions.

The Neuman Systems Model (NSM) provides both a utilitarian practice model for students and a respectful, caring framework for nursing education. The model "emphasizes the need to consider both the client's and the caregiver's perceptions of stressors ... and assumes that nursing goals are established effectively when negotiated with the client" (Fawcett, 1989, pp. 75-76). If we as nurse educators conceptualize nursing students as clients, that is, consumers of our products, then we are obliged to respond to our students' perceptions, negotiating goals and outcomes according to their needs as well as our own. By doing so, we indicate our respect for their rights and viewpoints just as Neuman's model honors clients' rights, values, and opinions. Neuman's precepts, although developed in the 1970s, are relevant to today's caring and empowering educational philosophies.

But after philosophical enlightenment, goes a Zen maxim, comes the laundry. How do we wash away the residue of objectivism that prevents effective incorporation of a caring nursing model such as Neuman's into clinical practice and nursing education? One powerful means might be through a reconsideration of the child of behaviorism, evaluation.

We must recognize that behavioral objectives do have applicability in nursing education. As a representation of minimal achievement levels, these objectives are conducive to skill training. However, even though they may be worthwhile in psychomotor skills laboratories, they "leave no room for the student's ... enculturation into the profession and introduction to the ways of identifying, classifying, and solving the problems of the discipline. They stifle creativity and provide rigid and restrictive guides for evaluation" (Bevis, 1989, p. 30). Bevis goes on to note that behaviorist evaluation models "undermine the educative-caring paradigm" (1989, p. 262) and proposes an evaluation model based on Stenhouse, Benner, and Eisner along with her own experience. Certainly, this model has its advantages with its shift of "teacher" to "co-learner" and "evaluation" to "criticism," which rests on trust. Bevis goes on to recommend Eisner's connoisseurship and criticism where power is shared, a position reflective of the curriculum revolution. This position of connoisseurship is naturalistic and artistic but still approaches evaluation from the standpoint of faculty.

A New Look at Evaluation, Caring, and the Neuman Systems Model

Belenky and colleagues (1986) trace the cognitive and ethical development of women in somewhat different terms than the development of men. (It is important to note that this framework of epistemological and ethical development, although more common among women, is also found in men.) According to these authors, most beginning college students occupy the position of "received knowers" who equate receiving knowledge with learning and believe that authorities are the ultimate source of truth. Even "multiplists," a more mature group of knowers, still believe that correct answers come from the teacher. But, often because of a failure of male authority, these knowers may turn inward, away from external authorities as their source of knowledge and begin to distrust logic, seeing "truth" as their own intuition.

Parallels are easily discovered between the work of Belenky and colleagues (1986) and Benner (1984). Benner's notion of a "novice" learner corresponds to Belenky and colleagues' "received knowing." Benner's dualistic thinkers display limited, inflexible, rule-governed behavior because they have no previous experience in nursing. The "advanced beginner," who corresponds to Belenky and colleagues' "multiplist," operates on guidelines developed by self or the instructor. This practitioner begins to perceive meaningful patterns but is unable to set priorities. They "can take in little of the situation: it is too new, too strange, and they still have to concentrate on remembering the rules they have been taught" (Benner, 1984, p. 24). This is the position of most new nursing graduates.

Clearly, this level of epistemological development will not solidly support professional expectations of the graduate nurses as flexible, independent problem-solvers capable of educating and leading clients toward wellness. Drawing upon Neuman's work (1995), we would say that we expect students to become skillful at deflecting stressors which assault their clients' lines of defense and at identifying client strengths as a basis for nursing intervention. In these days of curriculum revolution, faculty must be prepared to encourage students' incorporation of a practice model such as Neuman's in an atmosphere of trust, respect, and empowerment as we explore the world of nursing together.

Extending the Construct of Evaluation

With Bevis as a guide for revolutionary thinking, let us extend our examination of the construct of evaluation. Firstly, does the word itself connote an uncomfortable and adversarial relationship? If so, our meaning must be revised and clarified. The word we use to identify the process is probably unimportant so long as it is free of negative connotations, but one might choose the terms "progression," "evolution," "transition," or "passage." Or perhaps, the notion of progress toward desired outcomes could be called a clinical "journey," mirroring Nelm's (1991) ideas about curriculum as an educational journey through the culture of nursing. Whatever we call it, we must imply a collegial process based on empowerment and caring, calculated to promote growth while maintaining self-esteem and focused on context and education rather than behavioral objectives and indoctrination. For our purposes, let us name this process "clinical transition," reflecting our identified need for movement through increasingly mature levels of thinking and practice.

"More than two decades ago, Hilda Taba maintained that evaluation is a cooperative activity" (Ornstein & Hunkins, 1988, p. 273). In Taba's mind, cooperation of teachers, administrators, and evaluators was necessary so that the effects of the curriculum on students could be ascertained. However, the effect of engagement of students with faculty is not addressed in this behavioristic paradigm. If emancipation is the gift of education as Bevis (1989) says, then evaluation—our "clinical transition"—requires collaboration of student and faculty in the process. Therefore, let us look more closely at models that emancipate and empower students while providing clinical mentorship.

The Process at Yakima Valley Community College

Faculty concerns about needs for student empowerment and clinical efficacy guided curriculum revision in the Yakima Valley Community College (YVCC) Associate Degree Nursing Program. One approach chosen by the faculty to foster independent problem-solving allied with caring was a change in our clinical evaluation process. Various models of evaluation were explored. We settled on naturalistic evaluation as the approach most congruent with the nature of nursing and our Neuman-based program Statement of Beliefs. Naturalistic models are participant-oriented, protect cultural pluralism (a major concern in our ethnically diverse student body), and provide a more complete, more wholistic view of education as a complex human endeavor to be understood in context. These models can be more difficult to use in that they depend on inductive reasoning instead of the "cookbook" approach of behavioral objectives, but they supply substantial, descriptive data and record multiple realities. These data are factual and confirmable and reflect perspectives of both faculty and students.

Naturalistic models also tend to be more extensive because they are not restricted to a narrow spectrum of behaviors and are therefore more valuable in assisting student and faculty to see the true scope of success or error. In addition, these models flow from program activity rather than intent, an important consideration for outcome criteria necessary for accreditation. Because they are adaptable—that is, not constrained by a preordinate design—they mold themselves to a variety of clinical settings and program requirements. Although the models are sensitive to different value systems, they permit the use of supporting empirical methods when necessary—an important consideration for maintenance of rigor and program integrity. Participants also enjoy feedback in natural, unstilted language rather than the formalized statements of behavioral objectives. One of the most important attributes of these models is their ability to shift the locus of formal judgment from faculty to student (Worthen & Sanders, 1987), thereby promoting analytic thinking and problem-solving activity.

Guba and Lincoln's fourth-generation evaluation was selected as the most appropriate for our "clinical transition." In this process, the "claims, concerns, and issues of stakeholders serve as organizational foci (the basis for determining what information is needed)" (Guba & Lincoln, 1989, p. 50). These authors believe that stakeholders, or groups at risk, must all be heard and that they must be able to actually use the information generated to help themselves grow. Guba and Lincoln warn that, because evaluation generates information and information is power, it must be shared in order to avoid exploitation and disenfranchisement. They recommend that the scope of the process be broad enough to address participants' claims, concerns, and issues while requiring that each stakeholder take into account all other stakeholders' input.

Guba and Lincoln have much in common with Neuman. Their emphasis on the importance of wholistic, contextual evaluation of a broad spectrum of behaviors through an adaptable design mirrors Neuman's work. In addition, fourth-generation evaluation is applicable cross-culturally, as is Neuman's model. Both frameworks encourage qualitative or interpretive methodology buttressed by rigorous scientific objectivism, and both promote respect for stakeholders.

In summary, fourth-generation evaluation not only recognizes stakeholders, but it endorses the importance of context, permits evaluation on a situation-by-situation basis, and acknowledges values of participants as the root of the evaluative process. This process was adopted by the YVCC Nursing Program to serve as both a means and an end in measuring student progress. In other words, Guba and Lincoln's (1989) fourth-generation evaluation process (as displayed in **Table 12.1**) was utilized not only to construct a clinical evaluation tool for the new YVCC curriculum, but was also employed as a framework for future implementation of "clinical transition" activity.

The "Clinical Transition" Tool

The "clinical transition" tool that was eventually developed as a result of these discussions was surprisingly simple (**Figure 12.1**). It consists of three questions requiring independent problem-solving and critical thinking as a basis for student self-report. These questions furnish an opportunity for discernment between tasks done well and those done at a minimal level. Additionally, students reflect upon how these minimally acceptable actions

Table 12.1: Guba and Lincoln's Fourth-Generation Process As Applied to "Clinical Transition"

1. Stakeholders were identified.
Students and faculty from all six quarters of the nursing program were viewed as stakeholders. (In addition, previous interactions with health care providers in the community furnished data for the last stakeholder group, employing agencies.)

2. Claims, concerns, and issues about the evaluative process were solicited from stakeholders.
In preparation for an open-ended meeting with a faculty facilitator, students were asked to consider their experience with previous clinical evaluations in terms of these three questions:
   a. What evaluative processes resulted in good, positive learning experiences for you?
   b. What evaluative processes resulted in unfavorable experiences?
   c. How do you agree or disagree with the instructor's evaluation of you during those experiences?

3. Claims, concerns, and issues were critiqued and understood.
First, the thoughts generated by the three questions about evaluation were shared among students, quarter by quarter, and the faculty facilitator. Some students were openly hostile about their previous experiences. Intriguingly, many students who had been marginally successful in clinic felt unsupported and poorly guided by behavioral objectives while very successful students felt unrecognized for their clinical excellence. Concurrently, cross-fertilization of concerns from students in one quarter to students in another quarter was accomplished. In this way, all concerns were addressed and dealt with by all participants, including faculty who shared their concerns in a faculty meeting.

4. Consensus was generated regarding as many issues and concerns as possible.
Agreement about clinical evaluation was achieved among students and faculty on these concepts:
   a. Frequent, private, individualized feedback is necessary.
   b. Satisfactory/unsatisfactory rating is insufficient.
   c. Increased instructor availability is desirable.
   d. A compassionate instructor style increases student confidence.
   e. Behavioral objectives do not measure the scope of learning or provide clear expectations in all important areas.

5. Negotiate on items with incomplete or no consensus.
Although students desired more instructor-student time in evaluation, faculty were unable to identify ways to give students that time. Already supervising the maximum number of students in clinic, faculty could not promise to give additional time to lengthy evaluation conferences or written narrative evaluations. Faculty also feared the potential "looseness" of evaluation not based on behavioral objectives.

6. Provide information needed for further negotiation.
A literature review resulted in a synthesis of ideas about a potential evaluation format in which agreed-upon needs could be met for all stakeholders. In addition, the synthetic proposal addressed ways in which students would take the lead in narrative exploration of their own performance, while instructors could verify, clarify, or add to the student assessment, thereby lightening faculty writing load and sharing power. A list of criteria based on effective nursing actions in the clinical setting and suitable for leveling throughout the six quarters of the program gained initial acceptance from faculty as a "tightener," aimed at preventing ambiguous, incomplete evaluation.

7. Create a forum where negotiation can occur.
Sixth quarter students agreed to pilot the new "clinical transition" format while faculty solicited feedback from them about its usefulness and level of acceptance.

8. Provide reports on further consensus or concerns and issues.
Reports at faculty meetings kept instructors abreast of students' enthusiasm with the new process. Discussions of leveling continued and two additional criteria were added to the list. In the spirit of adaptability, faculty agreed that the basic list of criteria could be modified to meet student needs in each clinical course, although ordering of items would be consistent. In ongoing clinical conferences, sixth quarter students discussed with the faculty facilitator the advantages and disadvantages of the new tool.

Clinical Day #_____ Date _____
Student	Faculty

Student	Faculty
1. Discuss aspects of your performance in today's clinic that pleased you. (Be specific)	
2. If you could do today over again tomorrow, what things would you change? (Be specific)	
3. What information do you need to gather in order to make that change?	

Figure 12.1: The "clinical transition" tool completed by students at the end of each clinic session.

might be improved and prepare themselves to rectify errors at the subsequent clinical session. "Atypical" students are well-served by this format that places the knower solidly in the middle of the known. Their learning needs can be met through this tool with equity, in consideration of the students' sociocultural and spiritual background. The thinking process of students which underlies their clinical judgment and skill is the true issue at stake, and through fourth-generation evaluation, this entire process may be viewed wholistically instead of piece by narrow piece.

The faculty adds their own comments in the right-hand column opposite the student remarks on the left. These comments often provide suggestions for improvement and a brief validation of students' perceptions. They tend to be harder on themselves than faculty are! Both student and faculty comments are keyed to a list of criteria established for that clinical rotation (**Table 12.2**). These criteria support wholistic, wellness-oriented care (Neuman, 1989), focusing on students' ability to use the nursing process, think critically, demonstrate technical competence, and engage in professional, caring behavior.

For example, a student might note, "#1. I realized that I had contaminated my gloves immediately and was able to avoid contaminating the catheter as well." Faculty may reply to that criterion or refer to others in their comments. Not every criterion is addressed every clinical day, but by the end of the rotation all will have been considered. Because student and faculty have communicated each week about clinical performance, students always know where they stand. There is no need for lengthy mid-term or final conferences which use up student and faculty time and markedly increase stress.

A simple, one-page form, confirming success or inability to meet clinical expectations by the end of the rotation is completed for each student. If the student must repeat the rotation, a list of detailed expectations is attached.

There is no need for daily anecdotal notes on each student because daily comments are already made on students' self-reports. Faculty discovered that it is best to ask students to keep their reports in a spiral bound notebook so that none are lost. In cases where a significant clinical problem arises, faculty can easily photocopy pertinent self-reports in order to ensure documentation for themselves.

Faculty initially felt uneasy about the absence of specific behaviors for evaluation but gradually learned that every vital clinical skill or action was subsumed under one or more of the criteria. They feared their ability to delay advancement of a student when necessary might be compromised without behavioral objectives as a back-up. Instead, they discovered that a greater scope of observation and comment was possible. They also recognized that some students who had previously passed clinical courses under the behavioral evaluation system could not do so with the "transition" model. For example, some behaviors do not lend themselves to objectification, such as caring, moral commitment, insight, foresight, flexible strategizing, search

---

Table 12.2: Example of a List of Criteria Used as a Basis for "Clinical Transition"

List of Criteria: Quarter 6

1. Continually corrects errors in course of action; accepts responsibility, accountability.
2. Recognizes environmental cues and important aspects of clinical situations.
3. Interacts with clients and gives clear explanations.
4. Needs little or no prompting.
5. Demonstrates organizational ability, gaining speed in care.
6. Displays little or no hesitancy/independent/self-motivated.
7. Accesses information appropriately.
8. Uses sound clinical judgment.
9. Develops caring, therapeutic relationship.
10. Uses the nursing process to provide culture-sensitive, individualized care.
11. Works safely/uses good technique.
12. Records and reports accurately.
13. Provides wholistically for ADLs, basic needs.
14. Adapts care to condition and developmental level of client.
15. Seeks help and advice p.r.n./demonstrates collegiality.
16. Teaches/contracts/sets mutual goals with client.
17. Leads/delegates/works in groups/advocates for client.
18. Promotes health and coping.
19. Discharges responsibilities promptly.
20. Begins to set priorities appropriately.

for meaning, and a sense of personal and professional responsibility (Bevis, 1990). Although unrecognized by logical positivism and the scientific method, these characteristics are crucial for competent nurses. The list of criteria, however, does provide the flexibility needed for instructors to ensure clinical competence with both technical skills such as injections and cognitive skills such as critical thinking.

Relationship of "Clinical Transition" to the NSM

The NSM's underlying assumptions are easily applied to the "clinical transition" process. The lived experience of each student results in a unique personal system that functions according to its basic structure. Nursing students struggle to maintain the integrity of this basic structure in the face of constant academic stressors such as heavy reading assignments, unfamiliar clinical settings, and anxiety-producing examinations. The normal range of responses which they have evolved over time may, in the face of such assault, become unstable. Without intervention on the part of caring nurse educators, flexible lines of defense in these student systems may collapse. Through the use of "clinical transition," educators desensitize the "noxious stressor" of evaluation and prevent or minimize the degree of student reaction to invasion by "tension-producing stimuli" (Neuman, 1989, p. 21, 23). Frequent, constructive feedback focusing on growth allows students to construct their identity as nurses in a supportive, although exacting, relationship with a caring instructor.

Faculty can strengthen students' ability to manage stress through recognition of physiological, psychological, sociocultural, developmental, and spiritual variables which affect their flexible lines of defense. That is, acknowledging that a student's spiritual commitment to nursing, status in home and community, self-esteem, and feelings of safety may all be affected by what the teacher says and how he or she says it in an evaluative session can contribute to education with concurrent stabilization of the student's existing systems and their strengths. Nursing faculty can renew students' "available energy to support the system in its optimal state" (Neuman, 1989, p. 21) through caring, healing, educational environments which model caring, healing nursing practice. We can share our academic and personal energy with them as we function as co-learners and mentors.

Even failure to succeed in a course can be presented to the student as an opportunity for growth and eventual success. Faculty can work collaboratively as "gate-openers" rather than "gatekeepers" with students whose reaction to stress might otherwise prevent reconstitution. The Neuman model, with its focus on wellness and wholism, serves well with this view of nursing education and the curriculum revolution. In addition, its parsimony and flexibility, applied to students as clients, allows nursing programs to move forward toward contextual, caring education.

Currently, the National League for Nursing (NLN) attempts to determine prior to accreditation whether a program is actually *effective* in doing its job instead of whether the program is *capable* of doing it. The League will scrutinize carefully the list of criteria used for "clinical transition" and should easily recognize that it is derived directly from "characteristics of the graduate" set forth in the YVCC Nursing Program Implementation of the Statement of Beliefs. It will be clear to the NLN that the criteria provide a framework for observation of students' actual clinical activities and reflect overall desired outcomes of nursing education much more clearly than did fragmented behavioral objectives. It is a qualitative method, acceptable to the NLN, that uses the NSM to open a wholistic, caring window on the process of growth and transition in nursing.

"Clinical Transition" and Outcome Criteria

According to Neuman, the evaluation of outcomes during the nursing process either confirms goals or points toward their reformulation (Fawcett, 1989). In nursing curricula, the evaluation of outcome confirms or corrects the educational effort through provision of system feedback. For example, an educational objective addressing communication is found in the YVCC Nursing Program philosophy. That objective guides course outcomes, and from those outcomes unit objectives are derived. The successful completion of unit objectives which evolve directly from philosophical beliefs is measured by the student and faculty through use of clinical transition criteria (**Table 12.3**). The resulting measurement provides a tight feedback loop for curriculum evaluation and revision throughout all levels of the nursing program.

Table 12.3: Evaluation of Educational Objectives by Clinical Transition Criteria

Practice Course: Quarter Two of the YVCC Nursing Program

Educational Objective	Use communication skills effectively to promote quality of client care.
Course Outcome	Use and evaluate effective communication skills in the clinical setting.
Unit Objective	Utilize the nursing process for an operative client, focusing on the mental health concepts of fear and anxiety and the nurse's ability to use therapeutic communication skills.
Journal Self-Assessment of Clinical Performance	Clinical Transition Criteria: Utilizes therapeutic communication with clients/families and other health professionals. Records and reports accurately and in a timely manner. Teaches client.

In addition to evaluation of program outcomes, the clinical transition criteria furnish a template for assessment of student outcomes. As a result of the qualitative, as well as quantitative, power of the criteria, notions such as "the ability to behave flexibly" (Valiga, 1988, p. 184) can be considered during student assessment. In fact, Valiga's list of components of cognitive maturity is not unlike the criteria of "clinical transition" (**Table 12.1**) and could easily be used as a starting place for development of outcome criteria for any nursing program.

Conclusion

Wholistic fourth-generation evaluation can be effectively used to promote trust and respect between student and faculty in Neuman-based nursing programs. This evaluation scheme is congruent with "a curriculum-development model that makes legitimate and central the caring mandate" (Bevis, 1989, p. 357) and encourages humanization in schools of nursing. Educators who know Dr. Betty Neuman would pronounce this caring view of nursing education as consonant with her personal ethos and her wholistic theory of nursing.

Acceptable student performance levels as measured by clinical transition criteria should result in graduates who are able to meet or exceed expectations of employers. The crucial test of curriculum efficacy, of course, is whether these graduates can find jobs and keep them.

References

Belenky, M., Clinchy, B., Goldberger, N., & Tarule, J. (1986). **Women's ways of knowing**. New York: Basic Books.

Benner, P. (1984). **From novice to expert**. Menlo Park: Addison-Wesley.

Bevis, E. (1988). New directions for a new age. In **Curriculum revolution: Mandate for change** (pp. 27-52). New York: National League for Nursing.

Bevis, E. (1989). Illuminating the issues: Probing the past, a history of nursing curriculum development - the past shapes the present. In **Toward a caring curriculum: A new pedagogy for nursing** (pp. 130-36). New York: National League for Nursing.

Bevis, E. (1990). Has the revolution become the new religion? In **Curriculum revolution: Redefining the student-teacher relationship** (pp. 57-66). New York: National League for Nursing.

Fawcett, J. (1989). Analysis and evaluation of the Neuman Systems Model. In **Neuman Systems Model** (2nd ed., pp. 75-76). Norwalk, CT: Appleton & Lange.

Guba, E., & Lincoln, Y. (1989). **Fourth generation evaluation**. Newbury Park: Sage Publications.

Nelms, T. (1991). Has the curriculum revolution revolutionized the definition of curriculum? **Journal of Nursing Education, 30(1)**, 5-8.

Neuman, B. (1989). **Neuman Systems Model** (2nd ed.). Norwalk, CT: Appleton & Lange.

Neuman, B. (1995). **Neuman Systems Model** (3rd ed.). Norwalk, CT: Appleton & Lange.

Ornstein, A., & Hunkins, F. (1988). **Curriculum: Foundations, principles, and issues**. Englewood Cliffs: Prentice Hall.

Reilly, D., & Oermann, M. (1992). **Clinical teaching in nursing education** (2nd ed.). New York: National League for Nursing.

Valiga, T. (1988). Curriculum outcomes and cognitive development: New perspectives for nursing education. In **Curriculum revolution: Mandate for change** (pp. 177-200). New York: National League for Nursing.

Worthen, B., & Sanders, J. (1987). **Educational evaluation**. New York: Longman.

Chapter 13
Clinical Evaluation: The Heart of Clinical Performance
Victoria Strickland Seng

The Department of Nursing at the University of Tennessee at Martin (UT Martin) has had a Neuman-based baccalaureate curriculum since 1988. Faculty decided to base the curriculum on the Neuman Systems Model (NSM) because their philosophical assumptions were congruent with the Neuman concepts of wholism, systems theory, and client interaction. Faculty members designed didactic courses to introduce students to Neuman concepts and in clinical courses students' experiences reinforced the didactic content. Objectives drive the curriculum in that the purposes of educational activities are specified. This focus assumes significant importance in the clinical area where students are expected to gain mastery of skills and behaviors essential for baccalaureate graduates.

In this chapter, I will focus on how the use of Neuman-based clinical evaluation forms affect student learning.

Evaluation Instruments

The clinical nursing program is divided into three levels corresponding with the sophomore, junior, and senior years. The evaluation packet is designed for use throughout the program and consists of three clinical evaluation instruments: (a) the Clinical Evaluation form, (b) a Summary of Clinical Evaluation form, and (c) a Profile of Clinical Evaluations form. The Clinical Evaluation and Summary of Clinical Evaluation forms are changed with the program levels and reflect achievement expectations for each level. The Clinical Evaluation form consists of a 25-item instrument with four ratings ranked from Intradependency (optimal) through Unsatisfactory (failure). Each rating is defined for each item on the instrument. Faculty and students use the detailed form to evaluate the students' progress toward achieving the expected level of performance. General definitions for the four rating categories as adapted to the Neuman model appear in **Table 13.1**. A sample of the differences between the behavioral rating definitions for each level of the curriculum appears in **Table 13.2**. At the end of every semester, faculty summarize each student's cumulative behaviors, using the Summary of Clinical Evaluation form to record the ratings, anecdotal information to support the evaluation, and the student's responses. The Profile of Clinical Evaluations form documents student progress throughout the program. Faculty maintain this form during the program to demonstrate the individual student's progress in each of the 25 behaviors and to aid in the identification of patterns of behavior occurring over multiple courses. Further information about development of the instruments appears in the third edition of *The Neuman Systems Model* (Seng, 1995).

Table 13.1: Senior-Level Rating Category General Definitions

Intradependency (Optimal)	Satisfactory (Expected)	Dependency (Below Expected)	Unsatisfactory (Failure)
The student assumes the responsibility for his/her own actions within the functions of the nursing role and educational level of Nursing 400, recognizing personal strengths and limitations. Using the nursing process and synchronizing any interventions, the student initiates and provides nursing care in the primary, secondary, and/or tertiary preventive interventions to assist individuals/ families/ groups in accordance with physiological, psychological, sociocultural, developmental, and spiritual considerations to strengthen the flexible and normal lines of defense against the intra-, inter-, and extra-personal stressors of the environment and strengthen the line of resistance to promote an optimal level of wellness.	The student accepts the responsibility for his/her own actions within the functions of the nursing role and educational level of Nursing 400, recognizing personal strengths and limitations. Using the nursing process in consultation with the instructor, the student provides nursing care in the primary, secondary, and/or tertiary preventive interventions to assist individuals/ families/ groups in accordance with physiological, psychological, sociocultural, developmental, and spiritual considerations to strengthen the flexible and normal lines of defense against the intra-, inter-, and extra-personal stressors of the environment and strengthen the line of resistance to promote an optimal level of wellness.	The student, after discussion, recognizes the responsibility for his/her own actions within the functions of the nursing role and educational level of Nursing 400. Using the nursing process, with guidance, the student provides basic nursing care in the primary, secondary, and/or tertiary preventive interventions to assist individuals/families/ groups in accordance with physiological, psychological, sociocultural, developmental, and spiritual considerations to strengthen the flexible and normal lines of defense against the intra-, inter-, and extra-personal stressors of the environment and strengthen the line of resistance to promote an optimal level of wellness.	The student, despite discussion, does not recognize and/or accept the responsibility for his/her own actions within the functions of the nursing role and/or performs below the educational level of Nursing 400. The student provides basic care only as directed by other health care personnel.

Relationship Between the Instruments and the NSM

The clinical evaluation instruments display strong connections with the NSM both in conceptualization and in their terminology. Neuman (1995) began the discussion of her model by establishing its roots in systems theory. The evaluations use a systems approach and emphasize relationships with the client/client system and the health care system. For example, the second student behavior in the evaluation section of the instrument refers to documentation, and the satisfactory rating definition concludes with "after

Table 13.2: Sample Behavior Ratings by Level

Intervention - Individual/Family/Group Education

Initiates education/reeducation using therapeutic teaching principles and knowledge of client/client system's health state.

Intradependency (Optimal)	Satisfactory (Expected)	Dependency (Below Expected)	Unsatisfactory (Failure)
Level 1 Initiates education/ reeducation of the individual using therapeutic teaching principles for primary and secondary preventions and demonstrating knowledge of physiological variables; environment; and health state.	Initiates education/ re-education of the individual using therapeutic teaching principles and demonstrating knowledge of physiological variables; environment; and health state.	Performs with guidance individual teaching based on knowledge of common physiological variables and of health.	Provides minimal individual teaching needed for daily activities.
Level 2 Initiates education/ reeducation of the individual/family using therapeutic teaching principles for primary, secondary, and tertiary preventions and demonstrating knowledge of physiological, psychological, sociocultural, and spiritual variables; environment; and health state.	Initiates education/ reeducation of the individual/family using therapeutic teaching principles and demonstrating knowledge of physiological, psychological, sociocultural, and spiritual variables; environment; and health state.	Performs with guidance individual/family teaching based on knowledge of common physiological, psychological, sociocultural, and spiritual variables and of health.	Provides minimal individual/family teaching needed for daily activities.
Level 3 Initiates education/ reeducation of the individual/family/ group using therapeutic teaching principles for primary, secondary, and tertiary preventions and demonstrating knowledge of physiological, psychological, sociocultural, developmental, and spiritual variables; environment; and health state.	Initiates education/ reeducation of the individual/family/group using therapeutic teaching principles and demonstrating knowledge of physiological, psychological, sociocultural, developmental, and spiritual variables; environment; and health state.	Performs with guidance individual/family/ group teaching based on knowledge of common physiological, psychological, sociocultural, developmental, and spiritual variables and of health.	Provides minimal individual/family/ group teaching needed for daily activities.

significant changes in the individual/family/group's system." The behavior which follows focuses on reporting that data to an "appropriate member of the health care system." References to the client/client system as the individual, family, or group can be found throughout the instruments beginning with the first behavior under assessment—addressing therapeutic communication. The satisfactory rating includes the statement "Applies principles of therapeutic communication when gathering assessment data, reflecting knowledge of all factors influencing the perceptual field of the individual/family/group."

Neuman (1995) also emphasized "respect for the newer client-caregiver collaborative relationships." (p. 25) The collaborative nature of the model is evident in the nursing intervention behaviors as listed on the tool under "plan section." The satisfactory rating definition states, "Plans care with the individual/family/group and identifies supplies needed to retain, attain, and maintain optimal health, incorporating the health care regime." The model's wholistic and multidimensional approach to client care is also supported by the instruments. The intervention portion of the instruments begins by addressing client system care and includes the intradependency definition, "Implements wholistic nursing actions according to the priorities and planned primary, secondary, and tertiary preventions required by the individual/family/group and the therapeutic health care regime." The multidimensional approach is evident throughout the instruments in references to the physiological, psychological, sociocultural, developmental, and spiritual variables of the client/client system.

Neuman's (1982) discussion of environment encompassed internal and external forces which affect the client/client system, including intra-, inter-, and extra-personal stressors. She later expanded the concept of environment to include the created environment which consists of the conditions occurring in response to efforts by the client/client system to achieve wholeness and continuance without change (Neuman, 1989; 1995). The instruments concentrate primarily on stressors in the environment. The knowledge of client/client system under the assessment behavioral definition for the satisfactory rating begins "Develops a sufficient data base, using information from pertinent sources and including biographical data, stressors as perceived by the individual/family/group, and stressors as perceived by the caregiver." The definition concludes with a reference to the intra-, inter-, and extra-personal stressors.

Neuman (1995) defined health by placing it on a wellness-illness continuum and focused on retaining, attaining, and maintaining optimal levels of health through expenditures of energy. The instruments incorporate the continuum in behavioral definitions. For example, the Satisfactory rating for summarizing assessment information includes, "Discusses the client's current position on the wellness/illness continuum and identifies significant changes." In the implementation portion of the instruments, the Satisfactory rating is stated as, "The individual/family/group expenditure and conservation of energy ... to retain, attain, and maintain the individual/ family/group's optimal level of health."

Neuman (1995) conceptualized nursing as consisting of three levels of prevention as intervention. The evaluation instruments incorporate the modes of prevention as demonstrated earlier in the example provided for the discussion of the wholistic view of the client/client system.

Outcomes of Instrument Implementation

The clinical evaluation instruments assist students in implementing the NSM in their developing clinical practice and provide a framework for organizing their knowledge base in nursing. Faculty extend application of the model to the clinical evaluation process in that they view students as clients, thus using the Neuman framework in their teaching/learning role. The behavioral definitions allow opportunity for involving students in discussions of their performance and progress toward expected or optimal levels of functioning, thus emphasizing a collaborative approach to the teaching-learning process. Students and faculty have responded positively to the instruments. Both groups find the specific definitions for the ratings on each behavior helpful in achieving the learning objectives for the clinical area. New faculty note that the instruments clarify the objectives and student clinical behaviors improving their ability to effectively evaluate students.

The clinical evaluation instruments are also proving useful in preparing for National League for Nursing (NLN) reaccreditation. NLN's (1991) required outcome criteria related to critical thinking, communication, and therapeutic nursing interventions are addressed by the instruments. Each semester faculty use the instruments to focus on (a) Critical thinking, which occurs as they document students' development in the areas of reasoning, analysis, and decision making in nursing (criterion 1); (b) Communication, which is incorporated throughout the instruments through collection of assessment data, collaborative planning, implementation of care, and documentation and reporting care evaluation (criterion 2); and (c) Therapeutic nursing interventions, which show development of students' therapeutic nursing intervention abilities and serve as the overall focus of the clinical evaluation instruments (criterion 3). The students' progression in each of these three areas can be shown through the profile of clinical evaluation forms which provide clear documentation of the outcomes.

Faculty Development and Ongoing Evaluation of Use of the NSM

New faculty are taught the NSM and related evaluation instruments as a part of their orientation to the department and the program. As members of the teaching teams use the instruments each semester they recognize ways in which their teaching effectiveness is enhanced by use of the model, as well as questions or problems that arise. These observations prompt dialogue about didactic and clinical application of the model and lead to renewed commitment to the model as faculty recognize its effectiveness. Excitement often builds as new opportunities for application of the model are identified. Comments are referred to the department's curriculum committee which is charged with reviewing the curriculum and clinical evaluation tools each year and recommending changes as needed. Several changes have occurred in the clinical evaluation instruments as a result of the evaluation process.

Future Implications for Use of the NSM

Considerations of future use of the NSM in clinical evaluation include the potential for expansions in nursing education and nursing practice. Faculty at UT Martin are evaluating the curriculum in preparation for reaccreditation. They will be examining application of the Neuman Systems Model throughout the curriculum, and changes may be recommended in order to assure accurate explication of the model. As a part of that activity, the clinical evaluation instruments will be examined and revisions may result. Revisions could include greater involvement of students in self-evaluation and expansion of the behavioral definitions to reflect changes in the model.

In the area of nursing practice, as health care agencies have moved toward basing nursing care on the nursing models, several agencies in the region served by UT Martin have indicated interest in the Neuman Systems Model. Graduates from the baccalaureate program at the university have accepted positions in many of these agencies, and their knowledge of the NSM has been valuable. As the graduates assume management-level positions, they may design NSM-based forms to document nursing care. Clinical evaluation instruments may also serve as models for evaluation of staff.

Summary

Clinical evaluation instruments describing student behaviors defined in the terminology of the Neuman Systems Model and incorporating the model were described for baccalaureate nursing education programs. Use of the instruments benefits students by assisting them in mastering the model and by providing them with specific descriptions of the behaviors they need to employ in clinical settings. The model and instruments have potential uses in nursing education and practice.

References

National League for Nursing. (1991). **Criteria and guidelines for the evaluation of baccalaureate and higher degree programs in nursing**. New York: Author.

Neuman, B. (1982). The Neuman health-care systems model: A total approach to client care. In B. Neuman (Ed.), **The Neuman Systems Model: Application to nursing education and practice**. Norwalk, CT: Appleton-Century-Crofts.

Neuman, B. (1989). **The Neuman Systems Model**, (2nd ed.). Norwalk, CT: Appleton & Lange.

Neuman, B. (1995). **The Neuman Systems Model**, (3rd ed.). Norwalk, CT: Appleton & Lange.

Seng, V.S. (1995). **The Neuman Systems Model in clinical evaluation of students**. In B. Neuman (Ed.), The Neuman Systems Model (3rd ed.). Norwalk, CT: Appleton & Lange.

Chapter 14
NSM-Based Care as an NLN Program Evaluation Outcome
Barbara T. Freese and Carol J. Scales

Accreditation of nursing education programs by the National League for Nursing, Inc. (NLN) involves a process of program evaluation to ensure quality and accountability. This process is accomplished through self-evaluation and is verified through peer evaluation (NLN, 1996, Policies and Procedures, pp. 2-4). To provide structure and uniformity to the evaluation process, the National League for Nursing has established a set of 14 criteria for the accreditation of baccalaureate and higher degree programs. These criteria, revised in 1996, address mission and governance, faculty, students, curriculum, resources, and program effectiveness.

The Lander University School of Nursing has used the Neuman Systems Model (NSM) as the conceptual basis for its baccalaureate nursing program since 1982 and continues to integrate this model throughout the nursing education program. Lander's program was initially accredited by the NLN in 1988 and reaccredited in 1996. This chapter describes how the faculty incorporated evaluation of student use of the NSM into a comprehensive student assessment instrument, which will provide numeric, aggregate data for program evaluation.

Lander Contributions to the Neuman Systems Model

Lander University contributions to the development and promotion of the NSM illustrate significant commitment to the model by individual faculty and students, as well as by the School of Nursing as a whole. Two faculty, Professor Nahn Joo Chang and Dr. Barbara T. Freese, serve as Trustees of the Neuman Systems Model, Inc. Faculty have presented papers and posters at NSM Symposia, have contributed chapters to *The Neuman Systems Model* books (1989 and 1995), have made numerous presentations, and have contributed to other publications using the model. In addition, four faculty presented a workshop on application of the NSM in baccalaureate education at the Fifth International Neuman Systems Model Symposium in 1995. Students and graduates have used the Model as the theoretical basis for research and practice projects since the first baccalaureate courses were offered in 1985. These contributions by faculty and students were described in the Lander Self Study Report (1995) as one indicator of the program's use of the NSM as a mission-relevant outcome.

Curriculum Consultation and Revision

Following completion of the NLN reaccreditation process in 1996, nursing faculty have been engaged in curriculum reorganization and revision in response to changes that are occurring in health care. Under the guidance of consultant Dr. Fay Bower, one focus of this revision has been developing methodology and instruments to evaluate program outcomes, including the mission-relevant outcome that addresses use of the NSM as the program's conceptual base.

In the revised curriculum to be implemented in 1998, students will begin clinical nursing courses at the sophomore level; accordingly, use of the NSM for curriculum and instruction has been restructured as follows:

Level	Components
Sophomore	NSM terminology
	Wholistic perspective
	NSM-based assessment
	Cultural differences between nurse
	and client
Junior and Senior	All of the above

NLN Outcome Evaluation

The NLN criteria section on program effectiveness includes criteria that address program evaluation based on a written plan (Criterion 13) and address evaluation of outcomes (Criterion 14). The focus of this section is on the collection and use of trended aggregate data to make decisions regarding the effectiveness of the program in achieving specified outcomes.

Program evaluation outcomes identified by the League in Criterion 14 to be evaluated by all nursing programs include critical thinking, communication, therapeutic nursing interventions, graduation rates, and patterns of employment. In addition, the League requires nursing programs to identify two outcomes specific to their unique purpose for program evaluation.

Selected outcome criterion 14.8: Nursing unit defined. Under the 1996 NLN criteria, the Lander University School of Nursing has selected use of the Neuman Systems Model as one of two mission-specific outcomes to be included in ongoing program evaluation for reaccreditation by the NLN. Nursing faculty have defined this selected outcome criterion as "the ability of students in the School of Nursing to plan, deliver, and evaluate theory-based nursing care using the Neuman Systems Model" (*Self Study Report*, 1995, p. 137). Assessment of this outcome requires a methodology for determining the extent to which the program has been successful in attaining the desired outcome.

Program Evaluation Instrument

In order to obtain outcome data for evaluation of program effectiveness in achieving both required and mission-specific outcomes specified by NLN Criterion 14, faculty have developed a standardized clinical evaluation instrument to measure student performance on 11 standards that address the required and mission-specific outcomes of the Lander nursing program. Five standards address steps in the nursing process; the remaining six address communication, critical thinking, professionalism, research, leadership, and use of the Neuman Systems Model. The instrument also includes a section for course-specific standards. Student behaviors relevant to each standard are identified as indicators; faculty rate each student on each indicator using a scale ranging from 1 *(novice)* to 7 *(proficient)*. Results will be used to assess each student's individual performance in clinical courses.

As an adjunct to the student evaluation process, students themselves submit a daily clinical work sheet which includes all of the evaluated behaviors. Students record activities which they believe demonstrate the evaluation indicator, including the standard addressing the NSM. This self-evaluation adjunct further emphasizes the integration of the NSM into the clinical delivery of client care. Acting as a "mental check list," students are reminded that their nursing care has a theoretical basis.

Incorporating the NSM into program evaluation

Program effectiveness in achieving NLN Criterion 14.8 that addresses use of the NSM by students to plan and provide nursing care will be evaluated by examining aggregate data derived from the NSM standard section of the clinical evaluation instrument. This section includes student behaviors (indicators) that are evaluated by faculty such as:

1. Assesses client as a system in interaction with the environment.
2. Demonstrates a wholistic perspective on client care by incorporating physiological, psychological, sociocultural, developmental, and spiritual variables.
3. Distinguishes positive and negative stressors in assessing clients.
4. Incorporates nurse and client perspectives into care.
5. Uses the NSM to plan care for client systems at the level of individual, family, group, and community.
6. Uses primary, secondary, and/or tertiary prevention as appropriate.
7. Uses the NSM as a framework to plan care considering cultural differences of nurse and client.
8. Uses NSM terminology to assess clients and plan care. Course faculty will analyze each student's progress as the basis for his/her clinical performance evaluation. Findings will inform faculty which aspects of model application require strengthening in the individual courses.

For the purpose of program evaluation, data will be compiled on each of the 11 standards for each student graduating class at the conclusion of a designated senior level clinical course. Data will then be analyzed in aggregate form to determine program effectiveness in meeting each standard. Results will be used to make decisions regarding program effectiveness. This instrument is being pilot tested during the spring semester, 1997.

Closing the Loop

The cycle of program evaluation requires collection and analysis of data on program outcomes, evaluation of the effectiveness of methods and indicators used, and then making use of data for program evaluation decisions. The first set of aggregate data, collected in spring 1997, will be analyzed to determine program effectiveness. Aggregate data will be collected for at least 3 years to determine trends and to provide information for program evaluation decisions.

References

Lander Nursing Faculty. (1995). **Self Study Report For Reaccreditation Prepared for the National League for Nursing, Inc.** Available from authors.

National League for Nursing Accrediting Commission. (1996). **Program Evaluators' Manual: Baccalaureate and Higher Degree Nursing Programs**. New York: Author.

Chapter 15
Efficacy of the Neuman Systems Model as a Curriculum Framework: A Longitudinal Study
Lois W. Lowry

Many nurse educators support the notion that nursing curricula should be developed from conceptual frameworks. Some nursing programs select one nursing model to guide curriculum development, such as the Roy Adaptation Model (Boston College), Watson's Theory of Caring (University of Colorado), or the Neuman Systems Model (Neumann College, Aston, PA). Other nursing programs use an eclectic approach, combining concepts from more than one nursing model with concepts such as human development or human needs that are shared with other disciplines. In either case, there is little data to validate the efficacy of teaching nursing content from a specific conceptual framework. Indeed, effective evaluation is a key deficit in most educational systems (Worthen & Sanders, 1987). The purpose of this chapter is to present the findings from a 5-year study of graduates from a nursing program based on the Neuman Systems Model (NSM).

The NSM is widely used throughout the world as a framework for guiding the development of curricula, particularly at the baccalaureate level. Nursing programs leading to an associate degree are relatively new among model-based programs. Nursing faculty at Cecil Community College North East, Maryland, designed the first Associate in Arts degree program in the United States based upon the NSM. Faculty developed a sophisticated curriculum that serves well as a foundation for both technical nursing practice and further education at the baccalaureate level. A plan to evaluate the efficacy of a model-based curriculum was an important aspect of the curriculum design. The intent was to judge the educational effectiveness of using a nursing model, so that future curriculum decisions would be founded on sound data. The foresight and hard work of the faculty were rewarded by receiving unanimous approval by the National League for Nursing (NLN) for initial accreditation, retroactive for the first graduating class in 1983.

Faculty hypothesized that students who internalize wholistic model concepts will then practice from the model's perspective and will provide effective care to patients. Three research questions guided the study:

1. To what extent were model constructs internalized by graduates of the program?
2. To what extent was the model used in practice by graduates of the program?
3. What were the changes over time within and between classes in internalization and use of the model?

Review of Literature

To evaluate, according to the *Random House Dictionary* (1968), is "to determine the worth or value of something or to appraise." Within education the goal of evaluation is to provide systematic appraisal of the educational process, including the program, students, faculty, and graduates. Evaluating the success and progress of graduates provides feedback for the educational system illustrating how well the nursing program is preparing nurses to function within the health care system (Litwak, Linc, & Bower, 1985). Evaluation holds greater promise than any other approach in providing educators with the information they need to help improve educational practices (Worthen & Sanders, 1987).

Informal evaluation has always been a part of the decision-making process in education. However, the emphasis on formal evaluation as a conscious, purposeful activity was influenced primarily by the contributions of Tyler to behavioral-based educational systems. Evaluators who employ behavioral objectives as the basis for determining whether a curriculum or program is a success are referred to as Tylerian evaluators. Faculty in nursing programs, particularly, have espoused the Tylerian approach to education and are well known for the plethora of objectives from course to course culminating in terminal objectives for the programs. Successful completion of these objectives is tantamount to success in the program.

Another form of evaluation that has greatly influenced the progression of nursing is the accreditation phenomenon. In the accreditation process, resources, faculty, facilities, and appropriateness of program design were evaluated rather than the educational status of graduates. Although there are many accrediting bodies, the NLN has been the primary accrediting agency to set the standards for nursing education programs. In the late 1970s, the NLN mandated that nursing programs be based on a philosophy or nursing model. More recently the need to evaluate value, standards, and outcomes of curricula has led to the development of a plethora of evaluation articles and books that provide new approaches to evaluation (Worthen & Sanders, 1987). A characteristic of curriculum evaluation in nursing is emphasis on outcomes.

Evaluation research studies usually lack replicability because the program being studied is dynamic and is taking place in a naturalistic setting (Talmadge, 1982, p. 594). Thus, it is important to distinguish evaluation from experimental research. An evaluation gives up the opportunity to manipulate and control in order to increase relevance to the immediate situation (Worthen & Sanders, 1987). Evaluation can lead to decisions concerning program continuation or revision. This evaluation study was designed to provide data over a 5-year period that could assist faculty in deciding the efficacy of using the NSM as the curriculum framework.

Method

Design. The recurrent institutional cycle design (Campbell & Stanley, 1963) was selected for this study because it is appropriate in situations in which a given aspect of an institutional process is being presented to new groups of respondents on a recurrent basis. The fact that the experimental variable (the nursing model) was being presented to each new class made possible some degree of control. **Table 15.1** shows the design for the five classes, 1985 through 1989. Each class was tested at two points in time, 3 weeks before and 7 months after graduation for a within-class comparison. This time-series design controlled for testing, instrumentation, regression, selection, and interaction.

Second, between-class comparisons of both pre- and post-tests—separate sample comparison—controlled for history and maturation. Finally, two groups tested before being exposed to the model were compared to two groups who had been exposed to the model at the same point in time. This comparison controlled for history, instrumentation, and interaction of testing X. Thus, this design assisted in controlling for rival hypotheses.

Sample. The target population included all 128 graduates from the five classes—1985 through 1989. The study sample was 104; 24 graduates who did not return the questionnaire following graduation were dropped from the study. All except five subjects were women; ages of all subjects ranged from 18 to 55, with a mean age of 28 years.

Instrument. The instrument is a self-report questionnaire of 90 items constructed by the dean of the nursing program and one faculty member from Cecil Community College and is referred to as the Lowry-Jopp Neuman Model Evaluation Instrument (LJNMEI). The instrument is divided into two sections; the first includes five concepts: person, stressors, wellness, nursing, and nursing process; and the second section includes the four roles of an associate-degree prepared nurse: care provider, communicator, teacher, and member of the profession. There are 44 items in section one, each describing or defining some characteristic of the concept as defined by Neuman. For example, "I view persons as wholistic beings" is an item under the concept "person," and "I evaluate stressors that affect a client's normal line of defense" illustrates an item under the concept "stressors."

Table 15.1: Recurrent institutional cycle design

Class				Observations						
	4/85	11/85	4/86	11/86	4/87	11/87	4/88	11/88	4/89	11/89
1985	X	01	02							
1986		X	03	04a						
1987				X	05	06a				
1988				07a	X		08	09		
1989						010a	X		011	012

NOTE:
X = Program of Study
0 = Observations
a = Two groups exposed to model (04 and 06) are compared to two groups not yet exposed (07 and 010) at the same point in time.

Forty-six items are included in section two that describe actions a graduate may take when using the model in practice. For example, two items under the care provider role are "The Neuman Systems Model serves as a checklist to encourage thoroughness in providing client care" and "I use the Neuman Model in assessing persons according to the five variables." Respondents are directed to select from a five-point Likert scale the response that best describes their perception of a model construct or its use in practice. The Likert scale ranges from zero (never) to four (always), so that a mean score of four in each subsection indicates absolute agreement with the NSM definitions of the concepts and consistent use of the model in practice. The instrument in its entirety is published in *The Neuman Systems Model*, 3rd ed. (1995) on pages 209-214.

Content validity and reliability of the instrument were established before beginning the study. For detailed information about the process of instrument development and validation, refer to the chapter by Lowry and Jopp in *Conceptual Models for Nursing Practice* (1989).

Procedure. Three weeks before graduation all students from the graduating class were asked to complete the questionnaire. Students were asked to give their permission to participate in the study by signing a cover letter. Anonymity was assured by assigning each questionnaire an identification number. No student refused to complete the questionnaire at this first testing. The nature of the study had been explained to students and they enthusiastically supported the project. Seven months following graduation the questionnaire was mailed to each graduate for the second testing with a cover letter requesting that the student complete and return the instrument. If graduates did not respond in 3 weeks, a reminder post card was sent. Response rates for the second questionnaire were between 50% and 60% for the first three classes and 15% for the last two classes. The dean and faculty member who designed the study had left the institution at the end of the third year of the study which may have influenced the poor return rates for 1988 and 1989.

Findings

Frequencies were calculated for each of the nine subscales at the time of graduation and 7 months later for all students from the classes of 1985 through 1989. The classes of 1988 and 1989, who completed the instrument on their first day of class, were the control groups. **Tables 15.2** and **15.3** show the grand means for the subsets of constructs. At the time of graduation, students reported most of the time that they perceived persons as wholistic beings (class means ranged from 3.16 to 3.71 on a 4-point scale).

Seven months after graduation the grand mean scores were comparable (class means ranged from 3.16 to 3.51), indicating that students' perceptions of person had changed very little over time. Likewise, students' perceptions of the goals of the three preventions as intervention were found to be well understood, with comparable overall means at graduation (class

Table 15.2: Perception of Neuman Model Constructs by all Classes

Construct	Control (n = 49) M	Graduation (n = 84) M	7 months later (n = 67) M
Person	2.50	3.36	3.37
Stressors	2.92	3.18	3.27
Wellness	3.08	3.19	3.32
Prevention as Intervention	2.82	3.21	3.30
Nursing Process	2.95	3.19	3.20

ranges 2.88-3.51) and after 7 months of practice (class ranges 3.04-3.49). Students also indicated both at graduation and 7 months later, that they used the nursing process most of the time. Of the items characterizing attributes of the construct "Prevention as Intervention" those that received the highest mean scores were: (a) assisting clients to attain maximum wellness ($M = 3.53$) and (b) involving clients with their care ($M = 3.42$). The item with the lowest mean was involving the family with client care ($M = 3.04$).

Students reported assessing client perceptions of stressors and their effect on client stability most of the time both at graduation (class ranges 2.91-3.25) and 7 months later (class ranged 3.00-3.61). Students accepted Neuman's perception of health as wellness most of the time at graduation, with a slight increase in this perception 7 months later (class ranges 2.88-3.51 and 3.12-3.46, respectively). It is encouraging that the grand means for each construct increased over time, indicating greater internalization of the model as graduates continued in practice following graduation. All the control scores were considerably lower for each construct, with one exception. The construct "wellness" appeared to be widely understood at the "lay" level, indicating that the public understands the terms and definitions associated with the word "wellness."

Students' use of the model when fulfilling practice roles was not as evident as shown by the grand means shown in **Table 15.3**. As students evaluated their practice roles from a Neuman-based framework, the grand means of the five classes indicated that students used the model slightly more at the time of their graduation as they implemented the care-provider role than when they were in practice 7 months later. Class ranges were 2.66-3.51 at graduation and 2.62-3.34 later. The two items related to the provision of care which received positive evaluations were: using the five variables as a checklist for thorough assessment of clients and interpreting the meaning

Table 15.3: Use of the Neuman Model in Practice by all Classes

Practice Role	Control (n = 49) M	Graduation (n = 91) M	7 months later (n = 70) M
Care Provider	2.95	3.02	2.90
Communicator	2.67	2.85	2.80
Teacher	2.60	2.87	2.80
Member of Profession	2.30	1.89	1.46

of stress to clients. Following graduation, however, overall means showed a slight decrease in the use of the model when graduates provided care.

The variance among individual means within classes on all constructs was less at the time of graduation than 7 months later. There was more variability shown in the data for the teacher and communicator roles both before and after graduation. That is, graduates used the model less in their communicator and teacher roles 7 months after graduation. Interestingly, the class of 1989 indicated they were fulfilling the teacher role more than the other classes. Perhaps understanding the importance of this role had become more important as an effect of changes that were occurring in the health care system between 1985 and 1989 that required early discharge planning.

The frequencies associated with the member of the nursing profession role were the most disappointing. Grand means at the two times indicated that the graduates rarely experienced encouragement by colleagues to articulate or use the model in practice, either at the time of graduation or 7 months later. The items in this subscale receiving the lowest means before and after were: collegial encouragement of the use of the model ($M = 1.69$ before to 1.29 after), administrative encouragement ($M = 1.41$ to 0.83), and colleagues' use of the model in their practice ($M = 1.27$ to 0.77). These means indicate that colleagues never or rarely used the model in their practice and did not encourage their peers to use one.

Paired t-tests of means within each class were conducted for each of the nine subscales, comparing graduation scores with scores 7 months later, using the Bonferroni adjustment to control for family-wise error. The return rate for the questionnaire mailed 7 months after graduation was 60% for the classes of 1985 and 1987, 50% for the class of 1986 and 15% for the classes of 1988 and 1989. With these higher rates, the findings from the first three class comparisons are likely to be more reliable than the findings from the last two classes. No statistically significant difference was noted over time in new graduates' perceptions of the NSM constructs within or between classes, nor was there a statistically significant difference over time in the use of the model in the care provider, communicator, or teacher roles. However, the member-of-profession role did show statistically significant change over time in a negative direction as shown in **Table 15.4**.

Discussion and Conclusions

Following a 2-year exposure to the NSM as the guiding framework for every course and clinical practicum in the curriculum, students had internalized the meanings of the constructs very well. Seven months after graduation, graduates were continuing to perceive and define persons, stressors, wellness, and nursing as interpreted through Neuman's worldview. These findings clearly indicate that the model had influenced student learning by providing a wholistic paradigm for understanding nursing. One student stated, "The Neuman model impressed me greatly. It was interesting how all the concepts involved in nursing seem to fit into it so neatly. It makes understanding easy to see it all laid out so clearly." Another student commented, "I don't think I ever thought about how interrelated the parts of my life were until it was presented in the Neuman Systems Model."

The NSM not only provided an organizing structure, concept definitions, and propositions but also provided a process for the practice of nursing. With today's knowledge explosion educators are seeking ways to emphasize critical thinking and clinical judgment to enhance learning processes rather than "filling the vessel with too much content."

Table 15.4: Paired t-test for Member of Profession Role by Class

Class	Graduation M	7 months later M	t	df	p*
1985	2.01	1.51	2.18	18	.043**
1986	1.64	1.22	3.46	15	.003**
1987	1.95	1.40	3.02	18	.007**
1988	2.37	1.47	2.23	5	NS
1989	1.60	1.97	0.65	4	NS

*p < .010 by Bonferroni adjustment

** statistically significant

The finding that all frequencies showed high mean scores, and all but one *t*-test showed no significant change over time, is positive, indicating that internalization and use of the model by graduates did not diminish over time. Content structured by the NSM's framework and delivered through a consistent educational process enabled students to learn for the long-term. This is the goal of education, to provide the tools for one's professional practice.

When socialization in the use of a model occurs early in the educational process, students are provided with foundational experience that can serve them well in practice and higher education levels. Study of principles of thinking and organization from a nursing model perspective at the associate level of nursing education is also valuable for baccalaureate education. Educators can validate the efficacy of model-based programs through evaluation studies. Data can then be used to determine necessary revisions in programs to enhance learning.

The NSM, with its emphasis on viewing client systems wholistically, enables students to assess, plan, and evaluate care comprehensively, thus resulting in delivery of high-quality patient care. Some administrators, in their evaluations of graduates from the Cecil Community College program, have stated, "Send me more like her." Others have acknowledged the comprehensive charting done by graduates who regularly address the five variables and client's perceptions of their stressors. On more than one occasion, a graduate was asked to present an in-service program about the model for other staff members. The purpose of the program was not only to introduce staff to a nursing model but also to demonstrate its utility in providing high-quality care. These in-service programs were presented to critical care and pediatric nurses, showing the model's utility in complex care involving patients and families.

Work settings can have a negative effect on the use of models in practice. Most of these graduates involved in this study were employed in medium-sized community hospitals with a work force that had been educated before nursing models were introduced into curricula. New graduates should be encouraged to practice in the way they were taught—not to be discouraged when they meet resistance to new ideas in the workplace. The "we've always done it this way" attitude can have a devastating effect on new graduates, impeding the improvement of patient care and advancement of nursing. Colleagues and administrators are encouraged to support new graduates in sharing their ideas and insights. Increased collaboration between the educational institutions and health care agencies would decrease the disparity between the "ideal" world of academia and the "real" world of practice.

Nursing models are useful in professional practice. They provide an essential theoretical foundation for the entire profession, enabling nurses to be articulate about the practice and discipline of nursing. Models provide a worldview that enables understanding of the concepts of the metaparadigm of nursing. Nurses who learn to practice from this perspective will be able to provide excellent care for clients, families, and communities to advance the profession of nursing.

References

Campbell, D.T., & Stanley, J.C. (1963). **Experimental and quasi-experimental designs for research**. Chicago: Rand McNally.

Litwak, L., Linc, L., & Bower, D. (1985). **Evaluation in nursing: Principles and practice**. (Publication No. 15-1976). New York: National League for Nursing.

Lowry, L.W., & Jopp, M. (1989). An evaluation instrument for assessing an associate degree curriculum. In J. Riehl-Sisca (Ed.), **Conceptual Models for Nursing Practice** (3rd ed.). Norwalk, CT: Appleton & Lange.

Neuman, B. (1995). **The Neuman Systems Model** (3rd ed.). Norwalk, CT: Appleton & Lange.

Random House Dictionary of the English Language (College Ed.). (1968). New York: Random House.

Talmadge, H. (1982). Evaluation of programs. In H.E. Mitzel (Ed.), **Encyclopedia of educational research** (5th ed.). New York: Free Press.

Worthen, B.R., & Sanders, J. (1987). **Educational evaluation**. New York: Longman.

Chapter 16
Evaluation Modalities for Assessing Student and Program Outcomes

Sarah J. Beckman, Sanna Boxley-Harges,
Cheryl Bruick-Sorge, and Judith Eichenauer

Ensuring the quality of higher education is a concern for all education systems in the United States and throughout the world. Nurse educators at Indiana University-Purdue University at Fort Wayne (IPFW) initiated a master plan for assessing outcomes of the associate degree nursing program in 1987. The assessment plan, revised in 1994, incorporates three areas of program outcomes assessment: internal interim assessment, internal assessment at exit, and external alumni and employer assessment. Assessment findings are used for program evaluation and program development.

This chapter will describe how three Neuman-based instruments are utilized in this program to demonstrate internal, student, and exit assessments. The "Nursing Assessment Guide" has been used since the late 1980s. The "Student Clinical Evaluation Tool" has been used for interim assessment throughout the program. The Lowry-Jopp Neuman Model Evaluation Instrument (LJNMEI) is used for assessing educational outcomes.

Neuman-Based Instruments for Measuring Outcomes in the Clinical Setting

The Nursing Assessment Guide and the Student Clinical Evaluation Tool were developed and are utilized for interim and exit assessment. The Neuman Systems Model (NSM) provides the organizing framework for client data collection in the Nursing Assessment Guide. This guide evolved from the assessment guide published by Dr. Betty Neuman in the first edition of *The Neuman Systems Model* (1982). Application and use of this tool with case scenarios is presented in Neuman's (1989) second edition. The assessment guide is a framework which directs data collection based on the five client variables and stressors that affect client stability. Neuman concepts are integrated within the nursing process format in the Student Clinical Evaluation Tool. The clinical evaluation tool directly assesses cognitive, psychomotor, and affective student outcomes.

The process of developing these instruments involved many hours of faculty effort. A subcommittee kept the entire faculty informed of the progress. During the time of development of each tool, there were multiple opportunities for faculty discussion, critique, and exchange of ideas. These conversations enhanced internalization of NSM ideas by faculty who could then apply them to practice situations. This step is critical for the successful implementation of a theory-based curriculum.

The first instrument, "The Nursing Assessment Guide," is designed to assist students in learning how to collect and organize client data. It is introduced in the first clinical nursing course and is consistently used in subsequent nursing courses. Faculty observe each student's ability to assess clients wholistically—emphasizing physiological, psychological, sociocultural, developmental, and spiritual variables. Further, students are assessed for their ability and accuracy in making decisions for inclusion of relevant data and exclusion of irrelevant data. Thinking and decision-making are further assessed for accuracy, relevancy, and significance—as students use their assessment data to diagnose, plan, implement, and evaluate client care.

The nursing assessment guide is divided into six sections which incorporate basic concepts of the Neuman Model. These sections are as follows:

I. Biographical Data
II. Health History
III. Stressors/Factors: Specific to Current Health Problem
IV. Intra-personal Stressors/Factors: Forces Within the Individual
V. Inter-personal Stressors/Factors: Forces Between Two or More Individuals
VI. Extra-personal Stressors/Factors: Forces Outside the Individual

An important addition to the assessment guide is a six page glossary, developed by the faculty to define and explain the terms, concepts, and examples used in the assessment guide. The glossary promotes consistency of language for students' use in completing the assessment guide. Faculty evaluate the degree of detail and completeness based on glossary definitions.

Evaluation of student performance in the clinical setting has been a challenge for nurse educators historically because of the difficulty in eliminating evaluator subjectivity. This challenge is even more pronounced in situations where there are multiple evaluators of the same student population as is found in programs that utilize both full-time and part-time clinical faculty. A second instrument, The Student Clinical Performance Evaluation Tool, was designed to enhance evaluator objectivity while controlling evaluator subjectivity. Central to the design of this evaluation tool was the leveling of student competencies and weighting of evaluation items.

Neuman's concepts form the basis for evaluation items that are then organized under the steps of the nursing process universally accepted by the nursing profession. The actual tool is two pages long and comprised of evaluation items that are written in Tylerian form as measurable, student-oriented behavioral objectives. Each objective measures student-oriented performance in nursing care interactions with clients and staff members. Performance is rated as inconsistent and unsafe, consistent and safe, or exceptional and safe. Student performance must be minimally consistent and safe in all categories to pass the clinical component of the course. A rating of inconsistent and unsafe in any category leads to failure of the course. An effort is made to increase objectivity by using a set of outcome criteria as a guide for the completion of the evaluation tool. For each evaluation item, the criteria provide a set of specific student activities or behaviors which identify whether and to what degree the objective has been met. Thus, through the use of these guidelines, evaluator subjectivity may be decreased or eliminated. Accompanying criteria for each objective are specifically written to meet the overall requirements of each clinical nursing course. Students use the same guidelines to evaluate themselves so that they remain aware of the status of their clinical performance.

Clinical performance abilities are leveled from course to course. Performance items become more numerous and increasingly complex from 100 to 200 level courses. Each evaluation item is weighted and operationally defined by criteria that identify specific clinical abilities and outcomes in order to differentiate clinical performance. **Table 16.1** displays a sample from the evaluation tool.

This Student Clinical Performance Evaluation Tool allows for easy introduction of additional evaluation items as needed. For example, following development and piloting of this evaluation tool, faculty identified the component of "beginning leadership" as being a necessary inclusion in the evaluation of student clinical performance at all levels. It was easy and efficient to add leadership items to the evaluation tool, thus demonstrating its adaptability.

Table 16.1: Sample of Clinical Objectives with Accompanying Outcome Criteria

Assess: Stressors affecting adaptation of clients in the clinical setting.
Identifies aspects of the client wholistically.

Exceptional/Safe	Consistent/Safe	Inconsistent/Unsafe
Identifies & correlates all 5 variables	Identifies & focuses primarily on physical & psychological variables	Identifies & focuses exclusively on physical variable

Implement: Nursing care that assists the client to reach maximum health potential.
Utilizes teaching/learning principles.

Exceptional/Safe	Consistent/Safe	Inconsistent/Unsafe
Identifies parents' learning needs: readiness to learn, developmental, & vocabulary level	Identifies parents' learning needs: readiness to learn & developmental level	Rarely recognizes parents' learning needs: does not assess readiness to learn
Develops basic teaching plan without assistance	Develops basic teaching plan with assistance	Develops primitive teaching plan
Teaches appropriate content without assistance	Teaches appropriate content with assistance	Needs assistance in identifying content

Neuman-Based Instrument at Exit and Post Graduation

The third assessment initiative at IPFW involves the revised LJNME instrument originally developed at Cecil Community College during the 1980s. Chapter 13 describes a longitudinal study, the first attempt to measure program outcomes from a Neuman-based curriculum. This chapter describes our replication study that examines outcomes at exit and 10 months after graduation from the IPFW program. Data has been collected on four graduating classes and alumni as of this writing and findings are presented, analyzed, and discussed in the following pages.

History. Preliminary efforts on this initiative started in 1990. Three faculty (Beckman, Bruick-Sorge, Eichenauer) from IPFW presented a paper at the 1990 biennial NSM International Symposium on the outcomes of using the two Neuman-based initiatives reported in the previous sections of this chapter (Nursing Assessment Guide and Student Clinical Evaluation Tool). Additional efforts were encouraged by Dr. Betty Neuman and the NSM Trustees to continue this scholarly work and add a component of program evaluation to determine efficacy of the Neuman model as a guiding framework for the curriculum.

The curriculum committee had many discussions about the challenges of attaining and measuring program outcomes appropriate for an associate degree nursing program. Up to this time, no formal means of evaluating outcomes were specifically related to the program's NSM-based curriculum. Beginning a year later, the National League for Nursing (NLN) criteria required program outcome evaluation.

In 1991, we obtained written permission from Cecil Community College to use the LJNME instrument for a replication study. The same research questions that guided the original study at Cecil Community College were asked in this investigation: 1. To what extent were the model constructs internalized by graduates? 2. To what extent was the model used in practice by graduates? 3. What were the changes over time between groups and within groups?

Instrument Revision. Consensus among the nursing faculty was that the LJNME instrument (89 items) targeted appropriate and desired concepts. For ease of use, however, faculty decided to make some revisions and format changes. Changes included printing the instrument using both sides of the paper, decreasing the margin space, and using "landscape" format. These changes resulted in a three-page instrument, whereas the original tool required eight pages. The five-point Likert scale was retained except that the rating "mostly" was changed to "usually." The highest rank order was given a score of 1 and the least a score of 5 to be consistent with other evaluation tools currently used in the program. The negatively stated items using words such as "limit" and "confuses" were rewritten using less pejorative wording such as "places limits" and "adds confusion." To promote a more logical flow of ideas, several items were reordered within designated sections. Repetitious words in each item were printed in bold letters as a prefix to multiple items in that subcategory. Category headings were likewise printed in bold type to facilitate reading. Six items in the original instrument that were repeated as a means of reliability testing were deleted. Demographic data were solicited for education and employment.

Six new items under the heading "Manager of Care—Beginning Leadership" were added in response to the changing role of associate degree graduates. As noted in the previous section, leadership characteristics were added to the clinical evaluation tool. These characteristics were to be evaluated when examining exit outcomes. The original LJNME instrument did not specifically categorize "leadership" variables. It should be noted that leadership specific to associate degree programs was not mentioned in the literature in the mid 1980s when the original tool was created. The NLN defines program outcomes in three areas: provider of care, manager of care, and member of the discipline. Manager of care outcomes are operationally defined in the beginning leadership objectives. Neuman model concepts are interpreted to include organizing, prioritizing, teaching clients or peers, and delivering or supervising care.

A computer score sheet was used for data collection, and *SAS System* software was used for statistical analysis. Through the use of the scan sheets, time required for computer data entry was decreased. Similar scoring forms are used for nursing exams, thus graduates are very familiar with the form.

Although the original LJNME instrument was tested for reliability and validity (Lowry & Jopp, 1989), the revised instruments required further testing. A panel of Neuman content experts determined high content validity of the revised items. Feedback from the pilot testing confirmed reliability of the new leadership items. Internal consistency of subsets was again measured using the Spearman-Brown split-half procedure; the alpha level was 0.84.

Recurrent Institutional Cycle Design. The recurrent institutional cycle design includes both December and May graduates in contrast to Cecil Community College that has only one graduating class per year—five classes in 5 years. Data were collected from four groups in 18 months, just before graduation—December 1992, May 1993, December 1993, and May 1994. The post-test was mailed to these graduates 10 months later. The revised instrument was pilot tested with the graduating class of May 1992. Data were tabulated and tentative findings encouraged continuation of the study.

Discussion of Findings. The target population included all graduates from the associate-degree program at IPFW from December 1992 to May 1994, totaling 181 graduates. The sample included 100% of new graduates and 33% of alumni. Older alumni responded in greater numbers than others surveyed. Graduates were mostly women (90%) and within the age range of 20-25 years (37%). More than half were employed at graduation and 95% were employed at the time of the post-test. Fifty-seven percent of the alumni respondents were pursuing a BSN degree. Detailed demographic data is displayed in **Table 16.2.**

Neuman concepts rated very positively (1.35-1.70) are those describing stress and stressors; five wholistic variables (physiological, psychological, sociocultural, developmental, and spiritual) related to the client; collaboration in assessment, data collection, and mutual goal setting; and secondary interventions that help people attain and maintain maximum wellness. Likewise, means calculated for over half of the items measuring application to practice were also relatively high—positive to strongly positive—indicating that alumni and graduates used the NSM to guide practice at graduation and months after. Items that showed significant changes over time are displayed in **Tables 16.3** through **16.6**. *T*-tests of means were conducted on all items within groups and between groups.

Negative responses from both graduates and alumni were related to professional role socialization and member of the discipline measurements. Responses indicated that neither graduates nor alumni respondents felt that head nurses were aware of the NSM. Also, respondents indicated that head nurses did not encourage the use of the model. On a more positive note, respondents indicated that they were not discouraged from using the model.

Table 16.2: Demographic Data

Item		Graduates %	Alumni %
Sex	Female	89.8	95.2
	Male	9.6	4.8
Age (in years)	20-25	36.7	23.8
	26-30	16.4	15.9
	31-35	18.6	15.9
	36-40	15.3	9.5
	>40	13.0	34.9
Education	Pursuing BSN	21.0	57.1
Employment	Nursing	53.2	95.2
Number hours worked per week	<16	41.0	1.6
	16.1-24	31.4	11.3
	24.1-32	13.3	27.4
	32.1-40	7.6	51.6
	>40	6.7	8.1
Type of agency employed	Acute care	66.3	70.0
	Long term care	15.4	15.0
	Home care	6.7	1.7
	Other	10.6	13.3
Number of clients agency serves	<150	22.4	33.3
	150-300	14.3	3.3
	300-450	12.2	8.3
	450-600	19.4	18.3
	>600	31.6	26.7

Table 16.3: Internalization of NSM Concepts

Item	Graduates		Alumni				
	M	SD	M	SD	t	df	p
IA Person							
**I view persons as closed systems	-0.86	1.14	-1.47	0.76	4.79	162	.0001
IB Stress/Stressors							
**As a nurse, I:							
identify client stressors	-1.33	0.65	1.64	0.52	-3.84	139	.0002
attempt to reduce stressors	1.29	0.71	1.61	0.61	-3.17	243	.0001
IC Wellness/Illness							
**As a nurse, I perceive							
clients as passive recipients	-0.50	1.25	-1.22	0.89	4.96	152	.0001
ID Nursing							
**As a nurse, I:							
believe nsg. focus is to follow orders	-0.12	1.21	-0.81	1.14	3.99	243	.0001
assist clients to maximum wellness	1.45	0.64	1.68	0.47	-3.05	147	.0027
provide care without assist	-0.99	1.01	-1.49	0.62	4.65	177	.0001
view clients as fragmented	-0.73	1.28	-1.42	1.07	3.88	241	.0001
aim to reduce client stress	1.17	0.71	1.37	0.61	-1.99	241	.0478
collaborate with client care	1.14	0.87	1.45	0.62	-3.14	156	.0020
involve client in planning	1.27	0.78	1.57	0.62	-3.15	129	.0020
utilize secondary interventions	1.32	0.65	1.53	0.56	-2.29	241	.0226
**I collaborate with clients							
in completing the assessment	1.30	0.82	1.70	0.59	-4.19	150	.0001

One very positive sign is that alumni respondents felt very comfortable sharing the NSM with colleagues at work.

The new subset, Manager of Care—Beginning Leadership, received positive responses by graduates and alumni. Three of the six items reflected changes over time. Statistically significant findings indicated that the NSM was useful in organizing assessment data. The NSM is also used as a guiding framework to prioritize intra-, inter-, and extra-personal stressors.

Implications, Trends, and Environmental Influences. The findings for this replication study support theory-based education in nursing. Students at the time of graduation and practicing nurses 10 months after graduation indicate that they continue to internalize concepts and increasingly apply many of these concepts to professional practice. The negative responses in the "member of the discipline" section emphasize the need for nursing faculty to be involved with educating staff and management in the practice setting. Students, graduates, and alumni of the program can also help influence attitudes and behaviors of colleagues by being articulate and proactive role models.

The LJMNE instrument is accepted as a valid and reliable survey tool. Both the original study at Cecil Community College and the replication study at IPFW provided reliability and validity data. Further, analysis of data from both studies show similar trends. Incidental environmental factors might have influenced some of the responses for this study; thus, it is important that they be discussed. The health care delivery milieu has been changing drastically in the 1990s. Multiple efforts from a variety of sources are being made to curb the escalating costs of health care. The number of positions for nurses has been sharply decreased in many hospitals. Positions held by RNs are being filled with less educated, less skilled, unlicensed personnel. The remaining RNs are expected to be managers of teams of care providers. The primary focus of associate degree education is to provide caregivers and nurses with beginning skills as managers of small groups of clients. There is limited time in associate programs to teach how to manage teams of care providers. Further, many graduates do not accept full time employment. Health care delivery is moving from acute care hospital settings to home, community, and long term care settings that require more independent decision-making. Any claim that 2 days with a team leader or charge nurse in the 200-level clinical courses adequately prepares an associate-degree graduate for this leadership role would be difficult to support.

Table 16.4: Graduate Application of the NSM

Item	Graduates		Alumni				
	M	SD	M	SD	t	df	p
IIA Provider of Care							
**NSM enables me to:							
be flexible in providing care	0.73	0.90	1.06	0.98	-2.48	241	.0137
interpret clinical situations	0.77	0.86	1.07	0.98	-2.26	238	.0243
place limits on flexibility	-0.56	1.08	-1.41	0.75	5.80	242	.0000
**The NSM:							
encourages thorough nursing care	0.57	1.05	0.84	0.81	-1.86	240	.0375
makes no difference in client care	-0.74	1.15	-1/39	0.97	4.00	242	.0001
provides framework for NCPs	0.93	0.87	1.22	0.91	-2.24	243	.0260
requires in-depth assessment	0.77	0.93	1.10	0.78	-2.43	246	.0158
**NSM enables me to improve:							
diagnostic skills	0.59	1.06	1.00	1.04	-2.70	244	.0075
observation skills	0.79	1.05	1.29	0.97	-3.29	243	.0012
performance skills	0.61	1.11	1.06	1.08	-2.86	110	.0051
**I utilize components of the NSM:							
five variables	0.09	0.96	1.19	0.97	-2.06	242	.0406
stressors	1.06	0.78	1.34	0.90	-2.32	242	.0209
degree of reaction	0.68	0.92	0.97	0.99	-2.10	244	.0363
reconstitution	0.84	0.88	1.11	0.99	-2.07	244	.0398

One positive response to the many pressures confronting nurses is for RNs to pursue additional formal education so that they are adequately prepared for leadership roles. Classes in the IPFW BS completion program have increased in size during the past 2 years. One required nursing class that is normally offered once a year had sufficient enrollment to be scheduled twice in 1995. Graduates of the associate program are advised to begin baccalaureate classes immediately after graduation. Many of those who begin employment never return to complete their BSN. An increasing number of pre-nursing students are seeking advisement for both the associate degree and the baccalaureate degree. These trends reflect reports in a 12/26/95 news release from the American Association of Colleges of Nursing that enrollments of RNs with associate degrees or hospital diplomas is up 2.6% over a year ago and graduations of returning RNs increased 6.2% over the previous year—the highest increase in 6 years.

One local hospital that actively hires graduates from IPFW recently adopted another nursing theory as their professional practice model, that of Imogene King. Faculty predict that graduates from IPFW will be able to generalize and apply their theory-based learning to the other theoretical framework. The situation may affect responses of future graduates to the LJNME instrument. The challenge to new graduates from a Neuman-based curriculum is to apply the broad concepts learned about relationships within this metaparadigm to the hospital King-based theoretical framework. Both models are based on systems theory. Both models emphasize Neuman's ideas of client-nurse perceptions and interactions and King's ideas of mutual goal attainment. Having received a sound theory-based education, graduates

Table 16.5: Graduate Application of the NSM (continued)

Item	Graduates		Alumni				
	M	SD	M	SD	t	df	p
IIB1 Communicator/Teacher (Client)							
**The NSM enables me to:							
provide consistent care	0.64	0.99	1.17	0.89	-3.78	243	.0002
promote negative client response	-0.69	1.04	-1.36	0.76	5.22	150	.0001
provide structure for							
teaching/learning	0.70	0.95	0.98	0.83	-2.11	243	.0361
IIB2 Communicator/Teacher (Self)							
**The NSM enables me to:							
categorize new information	0.64	0.98	0.92	0.89	-2.00	242	.0471
organize & analyze data	0.64	1.03	1.06	0.88	-2.88	241	.0042
add confusion to information	-0.50	1.14	-1.28	0.93	4.82	240	.0000
make no difference							
in communication	-0.28	1.16	-0.91	1.17	3.58	235	.0004
understand new information	0.53	0.99	0.84	0.85	-2.21	240	.0281
improve my communication	0.44	1.08	0.79	1.03	-2.21	240	.0279

Table 16.6: Graduate Application of Member of the Discipline Role

Item	Graduates		Alumni				
	M	SD	M	SD	t	df	p
IID Member of Discipline							
**As a nurse, I feel:							
I share NSM with colleagues	0.13	1.21	0.52	1.03	-2.24	238	.0262
Head nurse is aware I use NSM	-0.33	1.21	-0.69	1.00	-2.13	237	.0340
I am encouraged to use NSM	-0.48	1.26	-0.97	1.02	2.68	234	.0080
I use NSM to adapt to new responsibilities	0.50	1.22	0.50	1.14	-2.53	235	.0120
I am discouraged to use the NSM	-0.97	1.14	-1.44	0.86	2.90	229	.0011

should be able to transfer this learning to the new situation. This is one of the goals of theory-based education.

The implications of these assessment findings are many. Nurse educators, students, alumni, and colleagues in practice are challenged to communicate, collaborate, and mutually plan. More communication about the utility of theory-based practice is necessary. That new graduates need continuing support from peers to apply theoretical concepts learned in their formal education cannot be overemphasized. Alumni should be encouraged to talk about their perceptions. Their confidence in continuing to apply these internalized model constructs will grow only if nurtured by positive, corrective feedback from both peers and managers.

This replication study was worthwhile for making internal decisions on program outcomes. Others are encouraged to replicate this study and continue building on this new body of knowledge.

Utilization of Assessment Findings for Program Development

A vital stage in any assessment activity is utilization of the findings for ongoing curriculum development. Faculty responsible for designated clinical courses analyze and interpret data with input from associate, part-time clinical faculty. Sharing among faculty occurs during curriculum meetings. The first two initiatives (Nursing Assessment and the Clinical Evaluation Tool) have been in place for almost a decade and have enhanced teaching. There is unanimous support for continuing use of both the Nursing Assessment Guide and the Student Clinical Evaluation Tool as described in this chapter. Student learning is facilitated as evidenced by outcomes from the third initiative at the time of graduation. Alumni responses on the LJNME instrument indicate continuing internalization of Neuman concepts and application to practice. The third assessment initiative contributes significantly to the program's overall plan. The assessment plan includes ongoing discussions and decision-making by the associate degree in nursing (ADN) curriculum committee for program development and annual reports to the

University Assessment Council. The work of educational evaluation is continuous and vital to the ongoing success of the program. Findings to date indicate that a curriculum based on the NSM is understandable, useful, and applicable to practice by ADN students, graduates, and alumni.

References

Lowry, L., & Jopp, M. (1989). An evaluation instrument for assessing an associate degree nursing curriculum based on the Neuman Systems Model. In J. Riehl-Sisca & C. Roy (Eds.), **Conceptual Models for Nursing Practice**, pp. 73-85. Norwalk, CT: Appleton & Lange.

Neuman, B. (Ed.). (1989). **The Neuman Systems Model** (2nd ed.). Norwalk, CT: Appleton & Lange.

Neuman, B. (Ed.). (1982). **The Neuman Systems Model: Application to Nursing Education and Practice**. Norwalk, CT: Appleton-Century-Crofts.

Polit, D., & Hungler, B. (1983). **Nursing Research: Principles and Methods**. Philadelphia: J.B. Lippincott.

SAS System. (1989). Cary, NC: SAS Institute.

Chapter 17
Development and Renewal of Faculty for Neuman-Based Teaching
Lois W. Lowry, Cheryl Bruick-Sorge, Barbara T. Freese, and Rita Sutherland

Faculty who teach in model-based programs are challenged to accept and maintain dedication to the model. Appropriate orientation of new faculty is vital so that they "buy in" to the worldview espoused in the model. Faculty must immerse themselves in the model so that they are able to develop courses and course-ware reflecting the model's framework. Revitalization of seasoned faculty is also important for maintaining interest, enthusiasm, and consistency in all courses in the program. This chapter describes strategies used by educators from several Neuman-based programs to develop and renew their faculty.

Becoming Acquainted with the Model
A strategy that can be used by faculty who either want to initiate a Neuman-based program or to revise such a program to reflect the Neuman worldview is to engage Dr. Betty Neuman or one of the Neuman Systems Model Trustees as a consultant to their faculty. (Information about Neuman Systems Model Trustees and how to contact them is found in the Appendix.) Having an opportunity to meet the theorist and engage in conversation with her enables faculty to "pick the brain" of the person whose worldview is being explored. Dr. Neuman's style is to present the concepts of the model and the linkages among the concepts in common language illustrated by examples pertinent to everyday living. She discusses variables of client systems, their common characteristics, and the need to maintain system stability in order to achieve wellness. She describes the effect of stressors on client systems' lines of defense that may lead to illness and death. She emphasizes the importance of primary prevention to help clients maintain strong lines of defense. Even when secondary or tertiary prevention strategies are the first interventions initiated, nurses can always include primary prevention strategies to assure that clients maintain an adequate health state following the stressor invasion.

As faculty listen to a presentation about the model by its creator or a knowledgeable trustee, they can appreciate the breadth and comprehensiveness of the structure. They can contemplate how their specific content area fits into the framework and can be developed into courses. This introduction to the model and opportunity for discussion, contemplation, and question-and-answer sessions is vital. Appropriate time must be allotted for these endeavors as well as creation of a milieu that encourages faculty interaction. A retreat held before or after a regular semester is most conducive to successful accomplishment of this goal. Faculty need time to digest what they have heard and read, and they need time to be creative. Dr. Neuman both inspires and encourages creativity.

During the consultation period, it is critical that faculty have opportunities to share their own philosophies of nursing and nursing education so that there is a "meeting of the minds." Areas of disagreement must be discussed and decisions must be made about how to handle diverse points of view. The beauty of the model is that its breadth permits faculty to interpret the model propositions from their specific area of expertise—for example, medical-surgical, adult health, maternal, pediatric, and so on. The "buy-in" to a systems and wholistic perspective is vital to the success of model implementation.

As faculty work with the model constructs and definitions, they assume ownership of the model and begin to use it creatively. In fact, they must be creative in the development of their courses because the model is broad—not detailed; and general—not specific. Faculty must make decisions about content inclusion and placement as well as selection of appropriate teaching tools such as case studies, care plans, and evaluation tools that reflect precepts of the model.

The reality is, however, that not all faculty are enthusiastic about developing a model-based program and in many cases they have been successful teachers before use of models became a curriculum expectation. The key to success is team building, setting group goals, and developing a time line. Faculty interaction is critical so that group understanding occurs. Through interactions, trust can develop followed by mutuality of goals and ultimately, consensus building. A key factor in the process is to allocate sufficient time to accomplish goals. A supportive dean or director is critical to this process, as is the provision of off-campus sites for work groups—away from day-to-day interruptions. Small groups formed according to content or interest areas can work together, then present information to the whole group for "validation checks."

Strategies that were successful in the development of the curriculum at Cecil Community College are shown in **Table 17.1**. The Neuman Systems Model was the foundation for the original nursing curriculum; that is, newly hired faculty designed the first nursing curriculum in the college based upon Neuman. In this situation, faculty did not have to break down former "ways of doing things." They had a charge to develop a Neuman-based program, a supportive administrator, much encouragement to be creative, and time allotted for program development. Faculty were hired 3 months before admission of the first class of students. During that period, faculty studied the model, shared their learnings among each other, and received consultation from faculty at Neumann College—at that time, Our Lady of Angels College in Aston, PA—who had developed their baccalaureate program from a Neuman perspective. These intercollegiate discussions were invaluable in developing faculty who were in the process of "internalizing" model constructs. As other faculty were added to the core group of four in subsequent years, they received a 2-day orientation to the model and were "buddied" with one or more experienced faculty members to assist them in course development.

Maintaining Faculty Interest and Enthusiasm

Indiana University-Purdue University. Because the Neuman Systems Model is an integral component of the ADN program at Indiana University-Purdue University at Fort Wayne (IPFW), it is essential to stimulate enthusiastic use of the model as early as possible by new and part-time faculty. New faculty view a videotape developed by senior faculty that presents the model, shows applications, and includes a commentary by Dr. Rosalie Mirenda, a Neuman trustee. Faculty are encouraged to attend the session in which information about the model is presented to students in the first ADN clinical nursing course. A live demonstration of concepts of the model is an adjunct to the session. Faculty are invited to attend classes related to the model in the BSN program's nursing theories course. Senior faculty mentor new faculty by familiarizing new faculty with Neuman teaching tools used in each course and by assisting them in evaluating students' use of these tools. Mentoring has the added benefit of "recharging" the senior faculty.

Table 17.1: Strategies Leading to Successful Implementation of a Conceptual Model

- Review the literature about the model.
- Define the constructs of the model.
- Define the scope of the model for your program.
- Encourage faculty to choose areas of exploration and development in which they are most interested.
- Share willingly the responsibilities among faculty members.
- Provide opportunities for team-building and values-clarification.
- Set specific times for faculty work sessions.
- Select locations conducive to productivity and free from interruptions.
- Maintain an informal atmosphere at work sessions.
- Encourage creativity, risk-taking, and innovation.
- Eliminate "tunnel-vision" and criticism.
- Establish a written timetable for short- and long-term goals.
- Appoint one member to keep group interaction notes to review from session to session for providing continuity.
- Encourage faculty to keep "idea logs" for recording creative thoughts, strategies, and ideas.
- Establish networks with faculties from other institutions that utilize the model.
- Identify and contact resource persons assisting with research design and statistical analyses.
- Plan the research design.
- Plan for reliability and validity tests appropriate to the design.
- Plan the method of data collection.
- Analyze data and draw conclusions.

Source: Lowry, L.W., & Jopp, M.C. (1989). An evaluation instrument for assessing an associate degree nursing curriculum based on the Neuman Systems Model. In J. Riehl-Sisca (Ed.), *Conceptual Models for Nursing Practice (3rd ed.)*. Norwalk, CT: Appleton & Lange.

Keeping all faculty enthusiastic about the model is imperative. Attending or lecturing at the Neuman Systems Model International Symposium is an effective way to stay current and get "recharged." Enthusiasm is maintained through networking with other model users. The Neuman Trustees and Dr. Neuman herself are always helpful and encouraging to faculty and students in the areas of education, research, and publication.

At IPFW a core faculty group continues to promote interest by use of the model as a framework for curriculum development, one-to-one mentoring of other faculty, and role modeling through presentations, research, and publications. The core faculty were instrumental in writing a program assessment plan that includes survey research as an integral component for assessing outcomes.

Success breeds success. When you have a tool such as the NSM that works well for teaching and promoting learning then faculty will want to continue to use and internalize it. Hence the model motivates. The model provides a framework that describes nursing and what nurses do while advocating for the patient who is in need of heath care, whether secondary, primary, or tertiary. The model has proven utility. Ultimately, faculty members' involvement depends on their state of development, understanding, and internalization of the model.

Lander University. Before developing the initial BSN curriculum, several strategies helped faculty comprehend the model. Initially, an intensive educational process was organized and conducted to orient all faculty to the model and how it could be applied in nursing education. During the process of initially developing and later refining the new curriculum based on the model, Dr. Betty Neuman and Dr. Rosalie Mirenda served as consultants to conduct a workshop for faculty about the model and its applications in nursing education and practice. In addition, the whole faculty engaged in several curriculum work sessions to ensure that the new and developing program was congruent with the model or that variations were thought out carefully and justified.

The NSM has now been used at Lander for over a decade. As new members have joined the nursing faculty, several strategies have been used to orient these new members to the NSM and also to ensure integrity in use of the model by continuing faculty. For example:

- Orientation to the NSM is built into the new faculty orientation process.
- During curriculum meetings, experienced faculty describe their use of the NSM for consideration by all faculty.
- Four faculty presented a workshop on use of the model in baccalaureate education at the Fifth Neuman Systems Model Symposium. This workshop was also presented for faculty and will be presented again in the future as needed in response to faculty changes.
- In a recent year in which 40% of the faculty were new to Lander University, a faculty retreat was held off campus for 2 days to reconsider

the program's philosophical bases, including the conceptual framework which is based on the model.

- In preparation for our NLN program evaluation site visit, faculty—full time and part time—held a working luncheon with student representatives to "talk through" how the model is integrated and applied throughout the curriculum.
- A loose-leaf notebook of numerous references that analyze the NSM and describe its use in nursing education and practice is available for use by all faculty.
- New faculty are advised to develop a mentoring relationship with an experienced faculty member and seek consultation and advice from the mentor in relation to all aspects of teaching and advising, including use of the model.
- Faculty are encouraged to submit model-based projects for presentation at meetings, conferences, and workshops at all levels—including the NSM Symposia. Faculty development grant funds are provided by the university to support these presentations.
- Faculty serve as advisors to support students in their use of the model for student projects and presentations; through this advising process, faculty understanding of the model and its applications is strengthened.

Santa Fe Community College (SFCC). In learning and applying the NSM, the SFCC nursing faculty have benefited from a close association with Dr. Neuman. Her guidance in implementing the model as a framework for the curriculum has been invaluable. New faculty are given books on the model edited by Dr. Neuman (1982, 1995). A module is presented to new faculty and available to all faculty. The module explains how the NSM with its emphasis on primary prevention is a guide for teaching the curriculum. All faculty are given the opportunity to attend introductory lectures on the NSM in NP-I. New faculty are encouraged to be curriculum committee members for at least 1 year to understand how the model is used as a framework for individual courses and for integrating the entire curriculum. The Neuman Systems Model Trustees, Inc. and the SFCC Nursing Programs co-hosted the February 1995 Fifth Biennial International Neuman Systems Model Symposium in Orlando, Florida. Nine SFCC nursing faculty presented papers at the conference, another indicator of faculty commitment and expertise. All faculty have attended national or regional conferences on the model.

When SFCC nursing faculty are asked about the effect of the NSM on their own critical thinking, community service, and research—nearly all state that the organizational qualities of the model are a framework for analyzing and synthesizing information. Assessment of clients' needs is enhanced, they believe, because use of the model helps assure them that all pertinent areas are addressed. As one faculty stated, "I think the model has been instrumental in increasing my ability to think critically especially in the areas of assessment and evaluation, not only in nursing but in health care delivery in general. She mentioned that in her activities of community service, working with the homeless at the Salvation Army and as a volunteer, she is "always thinking in terms of stressors, especially in the sociological, psychological, and spiritual variables." Her concerns for clients, she says, focus on "primary prevention and strengthening the lines of defense."

Fawcett states that "conceptual models guide research by stating what phenomena make up the domain of inquiry and specifying methodological directives about how the domain is to be investigated" (Neuman, 1995). A SFCC faculty member agreed and stated that in the research process she found the NSM to be valuable in helping to identify the specific research question from her multidimensional health care interests. Still another faculty member explained that she found the model useful in identifying middle-range theories that described, explained, and predicted responses of adult clients in two different situations following primary prevention nursing interventions in hospital and home-care settings. The situations include clients who were at high risk for infection or had impaired physical mobility.

Conclusions

Faculty who have had opportunity to teach in Neuman-based programs over time have come to "believe in" the efficacy of the model to guide educational endeavors as evidenced by the information in this chapter. We emphasize, however, that faculty should be revitalized to maintain their interest and enthusiasm, so they can extend the model into new applications. Networking with other NSM faculty and taking part in the Biennial International Neuman Symposia are vital components in the renewal process.

References

Neuman, B. (1995). **The Neuman Systems Model** (3rd ed.). Norwalk, CT: Appleton & Lange.
Neuman, B. (1982). **The Neuman Systems Model: Application to Nursing Education and Practice**. Norwalk, CT: Appleton-Century-Crofts.

Chapter 18
Vision, Values, and Verities
Lois W. Lowry

This chapter revisits the vision and values of Betty Neuman that have been instrumental in bringing the Neuman Systems Model (NSM) to its current level of usefulness in guiding the development of nursing theory. The author presents the verities of the model that are relevant to nursing education and practice as we prepare for our future. The year 2000 is like a powerful magnet on humanity, reaching into the 1990s, amplifying emotions, accelerating change, and compelling us to reexamine ourselves, our values, and our institutions. Looking at the origins of the model can provide insights that enable us not only to evaluate our accomplishments but to plot a course with confidence. By so doing, scholars become aware of the beliefs, forces, and situations that influence the birth of new ideas. Original ideas are often molded and modified over time to better serve the purpose for which they were invented. One creative idea may spawn another in a synergistic burst of energy resulting in a whole new pattern of ideas useful for some new purpose. Other ideas may create a momentary flash of insight that may be temporary or faddish. The latter may not survive in the long run, thus should be discarded as situations change or new paradigms emerge that require different ways of looking at things.

Nurse educators are faced with incredible challenges as the 21st century approaches. Movement from hospital to community settings for clinical experiences forces new faculty-student configurations. The focus on health promotion and wellness requires a teaching approach that emphasizes client strengths rather than problems. Illness care occurs in short segments demanding thinking about discharge planning with ill clients and their families immediately upon—and sometimes before—admission to the hospital. The teaching of families and the provision of care in the home challenges educators to prepare students in different ways to meet new demands. The knowledge explosion and complexity of health-related problems stimulates educators to organize content and process to better prepare students to function as nurse professionals in a rapidly changing health care system.

What educational models will embody the vision, values, and verities that are needed to prepare our graduates for these challenges? This author argues that despite changes in the delivery of health care, the process of information, and the complexity of knowledge, the NSM is an appropriate theoretical framework for education for the future. The model is sufficiently sophisticated, comprehensive, and flexible to embrace changes in content and technology without jeopardizing the model's integrity. A look back and then forward will validate this perception.

A View Backward

In the past 100 years, we have witnessed the evolution of nursing education from learning through apprenticeship training to the present sophisticated educational programs undergirded by theory, philosophy, and research methods. The discipline of nursing has moved through several stages of knowledge development on the way to scholarly maturity. Central to every stage, however, is the mission of nursing to provide care, enhance healing, and create an environment supportive to human health and well-being. Inexorably intertwined with the practice mission is the educational mission to develop curricula that can prepare nurses to function as generalists or as advanced practitioners within an ever-changing healthcare system. Regardless of educational level, assumptions about the wholeness of human beings, their environmental context, and nurses' responsibility to provide comprehensive care have influenced the content of educational programs. In the 1960s the focus on theory development led to attempts to identify the structure of theory and to define, explain, and analyze theory components. This trend was endorsed by the National League for Nursing's mandate in the 1970s for a theory-based curriculum as a criterion for accreditation. The milieu of the 1960s was the context within which Betty Neuman developed the NSM.

In the role of professor, Dr. Neuman's mission was to provide a unified structure for graduate-student learning (Neuman, 1995, p. 674). Students requested a program entry class that would provide an overview of the four variables of man: physiological, psychological, sociocultural, and developmental, which they would subsequently study in depth in clinical specialty programs. Guest speakers presented content within their respective areas of expertise in the course, thus acknowledging the interdisciplinary nature of the theoretical foundations of nursing. Still needed, however, was a structure that integrated diverse content into a nursing perspective that would guide both the study and practice of nursing. Neuman's own basic philosophy of "helping each other live" and her knowledge of systems, human behavior, theories of stress, and reaction to stress led her to develop the NSM within a wholistic systems perspective. Caplan's levels of preventions that are consistent with systems thinking provided the typology for nursing interventions. Neuman's own clinical experiences and observations in teaching and practice added credibility to the firm theoretical underpinnings (Neuman, 1995).

An article published in *Nursing Research,* in 1972, presented the model and a 2-year evaluation of the model's positive effect on student learning (Neuman & Young, 1972). Although designed as a "teaching aid," the breadth and comprehensiveness of the work attracted the attention of colleagues in education who were searching for frameworks to guide curriculum development in academic nursing. The NLN mandate for theory-based curricula heightened awareness of the significance of theory for both education and practice. Concomitantly, systems theory was increasingly an accepted framework in the disciplines of biology, engineering, business, organizations, and family psychoanalysis, thus demonstrating its interdisciplinary versatility and applicability. Educators, sensitive to the trends and dedicated to student learning, sought guidance about nursing models from Reihl's (1974) book *Conceptual Models for Nursing Practice*. One chapter devoted to the Neuman Health Care Systems Model classified the framework as a systems model. Nurse educators who adopted the model quickly discovered the utility of systems thinking for curriculum development and student learning. Neuman consulted with interested schools to assist them in interpreting the model constructs and providing direction for the development of model-based curricula.

Neuman's original model is based on assumptions about people as wholistic beings—unique, yet similar—whose equilibrium can be disturbed by both internal and external stressors. Neuman also assumes that individuals develop a range of responses over time that may assist them in cushioning the blows of stressors in an attempt to stabilize their equilibrium so that health is maintained (Neuman & Young, 1972). In other words, people and their environments are in dynamic interaction sustained by energy that can preserve and enhance system integrity. If energy becomes depleted, illness occurs and the system becomes unstable. The goal is for the system to maintain stability. The health provider's role is to support linkages among people, their environment, and their health states so that the system remains stable and optimal health is attained, regained, or maintained.

These assumptions were the basic principles that undergirded model development. Educators who choose the model to structure a nursing curriculum first must accept these assumptions, then proceed to develop courses from a model perspective. The model provides the framework; the assumptions determine the world view. A look into the past illustrates how Neuman's vision enabled development of a model that was successful for curriculum development.

Twenty-five years later as educators consider present and future nursing education programs they must reflect on values and verities needed to guide future nursing curriculum development. They must reinforce universal truths and consider eliminating obsolete information. The future demands relevance, parsimony, critical thinking, humanism, cost effectiveness, continuous quality improvement, and a global perspective. Do Neuman's assumptions of yesterday provide universal values that are relevant for the demands of tomorrow? A consideration of current trends can help us answer these questions.

A View Forward

One of the most exciting breakthroughs of the 21st century is the expanding concept of what it means to be human (Naisbitt & Aburdene, 1990). As our horizons widen and the globe "shrinks" we are placing greater value on individuals, their cultures, diversity, and contributions to our world. Goals of many groups are directed toward humanitarian issues such as the war on hunger and poverty, a drug-free society, cures for illness, and death with dignity. There is renewed interest in the spiritual dimension of personhood including a better understanding of body, mind, and spirit connections. An interest in and practice of religious beliefs is intensifying worldwide. People are reaffirming the spiritual as a more balanced quest to better their lives. Religious conservatives and liberals alike are seeking links between their everyday lives and the transcendent. A New-Age spokesperson has said, "People want a living experience of spirituality. They yearn to get in touch with the soul" (Naisbitt & Aburdene, 1990). Neuman's first assumption values the importance of individuals. People are central to Neuman's model, whether defined as individuals, families, or communities. People are composites of physical, psychological, sociocultural, developmental, and spiritual variables that interface and influence positive and negative functioning.

Neuman acknowledges and promotes the spiritual variable as an innate component of people that permeates all other variables. The spirit controls the mind and the mind consciously or unconsciously controls the body (Neuman, 1995, p. 48). The more spiritually attuned people are, the more likely they are to maintain optimal system stability. More recently, Neuman (1995) proposed the concept of created environment as an individual's unconscious mobilization of all variables for the purpose of system integration and stability. One's created environment serves as a protective coping mechanism—for example, the more threatened one feels, the more energy will be needed to create a safe environment, and less energy will be available to function optimally. If, however, one's spirituality is nurtured and developed, then one has less need for the protective created environment (Lowry, 1995). The spirit empowers and in being empowered, energy is released not only for individual mental and physical well-being but also for humanitarian activities. Whereas Neuman's original assumptions about people remain relevant today, Neuman has provided greater understanding of people's psychosocial and spiritual connections. As Neuman's thinking has evolved, the model has also expanded. This underscores the fact that the original model was sufficiently broad and comprehensive so as to allow further development, interpretation, and refinement.

A second trend of the times is a shift from a scientific to a biotechnical model, for example, biology as metaphor suggests information-intensive, inner-directed, adaptive, wholistic (Naisbitt & Aburdene, 1990). Our world is in the process of creating elaborate information systems used to accelerate knowledge sharing. Humans must master the technology and learn to use information highways to advance and communicate knowledge. Naisbitt and Aburdene (1990) claim that humankind must evolve spiritually if we are expected to be responsible for life. Knowledge cannot be separated from human understanding, appreciation, and caring for other humans. Care and comfort have been the mission of nursing since early times. Interpreting, organizing, and communicating these attributes is the challenge of nurse education. Teaching ethics and ethical frameworks for decision-making has been a strong curriculum component since the Florence Nightingale Schools. Nurse education for tomorrow demands an even greater emphasis on ethics in our biotechnical world. Educators critically assess what information is essential in the curriculum and must teach and use computer technology to efficiently and effectively disseminate knowledge.

Neuman's systems perspective lends structure to our increasingly complex world of nursing practice and education. This perspective values wholes as well as parts of the whole and their interaction and influence on the whole. It provides a way of structuring information with a feedback loop for reevaluation of data. The cycles of input, process, and output comprise a dynamic organizational pattern that continuously moves toward differentiation and elaboration to promote future growth (Neuman, 1995). Databases derived from Neuman constructs are needed to further organize information that can be retrieved for research studies.

Nursing is viewed as being primarily concerned with identifying appropriate actions in stress-related situations that potentially or actually alter health states of people. Actions are derived after a thorough assessment of the client-environment situation, including clients' perceptions of the situation. This interactive and wholistic approach is dynamic and equally as appropriate for the year 2002 as it was in 1972. Perceptions and definitions of stressors may change from decade to decade, but the necessity to identify and implement coping strategies that will preserve the character of the system remains. Systems thinking encompasses human systems, information systems, and ethical systems. A marriage between high tech and high touch supported by a strong ethical foundation is critical to the education of nurses for the future. Neuman's model proposes caring caregiving in which nurses act to protect clients' own preferences, wants, and needs thus reinforcing links between human and ethical systems. Nurses practicing from Neuman perspectives will seek ways to protect clients' rights and to establish health policies that reflect social justice (Lowry, Walker, & Mirenda, 1995).

A third trend that is already having an effect on nursing education is the emergence of a global economy and lifestyle. Opportunities for travel, cultural exchanges, and advanced telecommunications among Europe, North America, and Asia encourage international sharing of ideas and curricula among nursing programs and professionals. Economic, educational, and cultural growth in Asian countries is coming into its own. Japan is leading the growth with South Korea, Taiwan, Hong Kong, and Singapore following close behind (Naisbitt & Aburdene, 1990). Economic growth is reinforced by each country's commitment to education. Not only do these countries send their bright and talented youth to the United States for higher education, they also have hosted international nursing theory conferences and requested faculty and student exchanges. Through cooperative ventures, nursing education programs can help the Asian countries advance their education and provide cultural opportunities for American students. Two nurse leaders of the national nurses' associations in Korea and Thailand were educated in the United States. They have taken the best of American nursing education as a prototype for establishing higher education opportunities and programs for nurses in their respective countries. They use nursing models and theories as the foundation for their educational programs.

During the summer of 1995, Korea held its first International Theory Conference that featured Dr. Betty Neuman as the keynote speaker. A few days later, Mahidol University in Bangkok sponsored its first Theory Conference that highlighted the NSM, and Japan also hosted an International Theory Conference, sponsored by Discovery International, Inc. Dr. Betty Neuman was one of three nurse theorists featured. The three invited theorists were selected by Japanese nurses as those whose contributions were most relevant to Japanese needs and wants. The relevance of Neuman's model is gaining acclaim in Asia as it has in Europe and Canada over the past 10 years.

Neuman's vision is and has been to extend the model to other countries. Beginning in the mid 1980s, Neuman was invited to present the model to audiences at international theory conferences in Canada, England, and Denmark. Advanced-practice nurses from Sweden, Denmark, and London invited articles and chapters by Neuman that presented primary prevention modalities in community settings. The Canadian provinces of Ontario and Manitoba adopted the model as the framework for the delivery of community health services in the early 1980s and continue to use the model today.

English is fast becoming the world's universal language as noted in areas of transportation and the media. Computer information highways also use English predominantly. Many Europeans are required to study English in school, thus can speak the language well. Asian countries are beginning to emphasize the study of English, although it is not yet required in the lower grades. Asian nurse graduates who return to their respective countries with advanced nursing degrees to become faculty continue to subscribe to American nursing journals to maintain their knowledge and expertise. This trend toward a universal language moves the world toward a global village. International exchanges in nursing can raise the standard of nursing education. Because the United States is a leader in the development of nursing services, nurses in other countries want to follow in our footsteps.

Dr. Neuman continues to consult for educational programs and practice settings in European countries, Puerto Rico, Australia, and New Zealand. In the summer of 1995, she visited five countries in Asia; and in 1996, she consulted in Kuwait. The trend toward using models to guide education, practice, and research is gaining momentum in Europe and Asia as educated nurses from these continents seek to develop a scientific basis for nursing. The NSM is appealing because of its breadth, wholistic approach, "user friendly" language, and emphasis on primary prevention—despite cultural and geographic differences.

During alternate years, an International Neuman Systems Model Symposium is held for Neuman scholars, educators, and practitioners so they may share their work among professional colleagues. Following the 1995 Symposium, international scholars expressed the need to develop Neuman-based handbooks in their respective languages. Contributors to these handbooks would present culturally sensitive case studies whose outcomes were Neuman-based. Culturally relevant examples would be used to teach nurses and students about the utility of Neuman's model. Franz Verberk from the Netherlands wrote the first handbook in Dutch to demonstrate the model's utility in social psychiatric nursing (B. Neuman, personal communication, June 1, 1996). Faculty from Chiang Mai University in Thailand are writing a monograph in the Thai language to be published in 1998.

Another exciting trend in American Nursing education is the emphasis on the delivery of nursing programs through distance-learning technology. Holy Names College and Kaiser Permanente of Northern California joined to sponsor a long-distance interactive Neuman-based video curriculum for their baccalaureate nursing program. Bowie State College in Maryland, another Neuman-based program has also ventured into distance learning that involves four schools! Today's technology is enabling the advancement of nursing education at an exponential rate and the Neuman model is keeping pace with the trend.

Neuman's original concept of a Health Care Systems model that would be useful for multiple disciplines is coming to fruition. East Tennessee State University uses the model as a basis for interdisciplinary teaching among nursing, medicine, family therapy, and social work (B. Neuman, personal communication, 1996). Likewise, at the University of South Florida, the model provides the framework for interdisciplinary team practice in rural areas among medicine, nursing, social work, and public health. The concepts of the NSM are readily understood by professionals from other disciplines who can embrace its world view. Sharing among disciplines that enables true understanding and appreciation to occur can elevate the level of trust among members of the interdisciplinary team. A trusting team collaborates in efforts to provide quality, cost effective care. Individual identity becomes less important as the team identity emerges working together toward this goal.

In the 21st century, nurse leaders are needed who possess wisdom and emotional integrity and who are committed to intelligent, cost effective, quality care. Educational programs must provide nurses with the tools they need to fulfill expanding roles in an ever-changing health care system. A comprehensive model can provide the structure from which sound educational processes evolve. The NSM is founded on values that are relevant today; its propositions contain lasting truths about people, stressors, and health. We educators who have developed courses and programs based upon the NSM celebrate the vision of Dr. Betty Neuman. We applaud those educators who have carried the vision forward and encourage others to take the model into the future. Dr. Neuman's vision is our legacy.

Vision without a task is but a dream,

A task without a vision is drudgery.

A task with vision is the hope of the world!

(Anonymous)

References

Lowry, L.W. (1995, February). **Spirituality and the created environment**. Paper presented at the Fifth International Biennial Neuman Systems Model Symposium, Orlando, FL.

Lowry, L.W., Walker, P.H., & Mirenda, R. (1995). Through the looking glass back to the future. In B. Neuman (Ed.), **The Neuman Systems Model** (3rd ed., pp. 63-76). Norwalk, CT: Appleton & Lange.

Naisbitt, J., & Aburdene, P. (1990). **Megatrends 2000**. New York: Avon.

Neuman, B. (1995). **The Neuman Systems Model** (3rd ed.). Norwalk, CT: Appleton & Lange.

Neuman, B., & Young, R.J. (1972). A model for teaching total person approach to patient's problems. **Nursing Research, 21**, 264-269.

Reihl, J.P. (1974). **Conceptual models for nursing practice**. Norwalk, CT: Appleton-Century-Crofts.

Appendix

The Neuman Systems Model Trustees, Inc.

The official mailing address for the organization is:
The Neuman Systems Model Trustees, Inc.
Neumann College
c/o Director of Library Media And Archives
One Neumann Drive
Aston, PA 19014

Mission and Purpose
The revised bylaws were approved 3/15/98; key sections appear below.

Mission: The Neuman Systems Model Trustees, Inc. is a nonprofit organization founded by Betty Neuman, PhD. Comprised of nurse researchers, educators, practitioners, and administrators, the trustees are dedicated to the ongoing process of supporting and promoting the Neuman Systems Model. Through a commitment to the future of the model, the trustees assure its integrity, development, and relevance to the continual enhancement of the body of nursing knowledge.

The purposes of the organization are as follows:
- Increase the understanding of the Neuman Systems Model within the nursing profession and the health care community;
- Conduct professional forums in which the professional community can be kept updated and apprised of the work related to the Neuman Systems Model;
- Maintain a bibliographic account of publications and research based on or utilizing the Neuman Systems Model;
- Respond to printed and spoken criticisms through intelligent and scholarly analysis of the work(s);
- Serve as consultants, advisors, and facilitators toward the ongoing development and utilization of the Neuman Systems Model;
- Support, through scholarly work and creative arts, the continued work and efforts of Betty Neuman, PhD.

Active Membership, Spring 1998

Betty Neuman, RN, PhD, FAAN
Founder/Director
Theorist, Author, Consultant,
and Counselor
P.O. Box 77, State Rd. 676
Beverly, OH 45787
Tel: (H) (614) 749-3322
(Fax) (614) 749-3322

Jan Russell, RN, PhD
President (1997-1999)
Associate Professor
School of Nursing
University of Missouri at Kansas City
2220 Holmes St.
Kansas City, MO 64108-2676
Tel: (W) (816) 235-1713
(Fax) (816) 235-1701
(H) (816) 322-8742
(E-mail) RussellJ@smtpgate.umkc.edu

Charlene Beynon, MScN
Assistant Director of Nursing
Middlesex-London Health Unit
Teaching Unit Program
50 King Street
London, Ontario N6A 5L7 Canada
Tel: (W) (519) 663-5317 x2484
(Fax) (519) 432-9430
(H) (519) 473-1743
(E-mail) cbeynon@julian.uwo.ca

Diane Breckenridge, RN, MSN
Post Doctoral Fellow
University of Pennsylvania
Abington Memorial Hospital
Abington, PA 19001
Tel: (W) (215) 898-0088
(Fax) (215) 836-2194
(H) (215) 836-2193
(E-mail) breckenr@pobox.upenn.edu

Barbara S. Cammuso, RNC, PhD
Assistant Professor
Fitchburg State College
6 Westport Drive
Shrewsbury, MA 01545
Tel: (W) (508) 845-9402
(Fax) (508) 845-9402
(H) (508) 842-3579
(E-mail) Bcammuso@msn.com

Cynthia Flynn Capers, RN, PhD
Professor and Dean
University of Akron
College of Nursing
Akron, OH 44325
Tel: (W) (330) 972-7552
(Fax) (330) 972-5737
(E-mail) capers@uakron.edu

Patricia Chadwick, RN, EdD
Vice President (1997-1999)
Professor and Dean
School of Nursing
University of Portland
5000 Willamette Boulevard
Portland, OR 97203-5798
Tel: (W) (503) 283-7233
(Fax) (503) 978-8042
(H) (503) 645-3741

Dorothy Craig, RN, MScN
Professor
Faculty of Nursing
University of Toronto
Ontario, M5S 1A1 Canada
Tel: (W) (416) 978-2857
(Fax) (416) 978-8222
(H) (416) 626-3529
(E-mail) dorothy.craig@utoronto.ca

Jacqueline Fawcett, RN, PhD
Professor
School of Nursing
University of Pennsylvania
Philadelphia, PA 19140
Tel: (W) (215) 898-8289
(Fax) (215) 573-7496
(H) (207) 832-7398
(E-mail) fawcett@pobox.upenn.edu

Barbara T. Freese, RN, EdD, FRCNA
Professor and Dean
School of Nursing
Lander University
Greenwood, SC 29649
Tel: (W) (864) 388-8337
(Fax) (864) 388-8890
(H) (864) 459-2626

Patricia Hinton-Walker, RN, PhD, FAAN
Former President (1995-1997)
Dean, Colorado University, SON
4200 E. Ninth Avenue Box C 288
Denver, CO 80262
Tel: (W) (303) 315-7754
(Fax) (303) 315-0076
(E-mail) patricia.walker@uchsc.edu

Margaret Louis, RN, PhD
Associate Professor
Department of Nursing
University of Nevada at Las Vegas
Las Vegas, NV 89154
Tel: (W) (702) 895-3812
(Fax) (702) 895-4807
(H) (702) 458-7792
(E-mail) louisrn@Nevada.edu

Lois W. Lowry, RN, DNSc
Former President (1993-1995)
Associate Professor
College of Nursing
University of South Florida
Tampa, Florida 33612-4799
Tel: (W) (813) 974-2191
(Fax) (813) 974-5418
(H) (813) 972-4011
(E-mail) doclowry@aol.com

Rae Jeanne Memmott, RN, MS
Associate Professor
College of Nursing
Brigham Young University
Provo, UT 84602
Tel: (W) (801) 378-7210
(Fax) (801) 378-3198
(H) (801) 225-1886   (E-mail) Rae_Jeanne_Memmott@BYU.edu

Rosalie M. Mirenda, RN, PhD
Former President (1988-1991)
President, Neumann College
Aston, PA 19014-1297
Tel: (W) (610) 558-5501
(Fax) (610) 558-5643
(H) (610) 565-2904
(E-mail) rmirenda@smtpgate.neumann.edu

Barbara Fulton Shambaugh, RN, EdD
President, Diogenes Ltd.
77 Pond Avenue # 1501
Brookline, MA 02146
Tel: (W) (617) 738-1500 x231
(Fax) (617) 731-0368
(H) (617) 566-6029
(E-mail) BJREADER@MSN.COM

Janet A. Sipple, RN, PhD
Former President, (1991-1993)
Professor
c/o St. Luke's School of Nursing
801 Ostrum Street
Bethlehem, PA 18015
Tel: (W) (610) 954-3440
(Fax) 610) 954-3412
(H) (610) 865-2003
(E-mail) 103226.2451@compuserve.com